YOUR
CHOLESTEROL
MATTERS

Also by Richard Furman, MD, FACS

Prescription for Life

YOUR
CHOLESTEROL
MATTERS

What Your Numbers Mean
and How You Can Improve Them

Richard Furman, MD, FACS

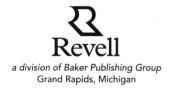

Revell
a division of Baker Publishing Group
Grand Rapids, Michigan

© 2017 by Richard Furman, MD, FACS

Published by Revell
a division of Baker Publishing Group
P.O. Box 6287, Grand Rapids, MI 49516-6287
www.revellbooks.com

Printed in the United States of America

Library of Congress Cataloging-in-Publication Data
Names: Furman, Richard, author.
Title: Your cholesterol matters : what your numbers mean and how you can improve them / Richard Furman, MD, FACS.
Description: Grand Rapids, MI : Revell, [2016] | Includes bibliographical references.
Identifiers: LCCN 2016032733 | ISBN 9780800728052 (pbk.)
Subjects: LCSH: Hypercholesteremia—Popular works. | Hypercholesteremia—Diet therapy—Popular works. | Low-cholesterol diet—Popular works.
Classification: LCC RC632.H83 F87 2016 | DDC 616.3/997—dc23
LC record available at https://lccn.loc.gov/2016032733

Unless otherwise indicated, Scripture quotations are from the Holy Bible, New International Version®. NIV®. Copyright © 1973, 1978, 1984, 2011 by Biblica, Inc.™ Used by permission of Zondervan. All rights reserved worldwide. www.zondervan.com

Scripture quotations labeled KJV are from the King James Version of the Bible.

This publication is intended to provide helpful and informative material on the subjects addressed. Readers should consult their personal health professionals before adopting any of the suggestions in this book or drawing inferences from it. The author and publisher expressly disclaim responsibility for any adverse effects arising from the use or application of the information contained in this book.

The author is represented by the literary agency of Wolgemuth & Associates, Inc.

17 18 19 20 21 22 23   7 6 5 4 3 2 1

Contents

PART 4: LIFESTYLE 3: EXERCISE

Preface

My quest to help people get healthy all began when I realized I was treating patients' symptoms, but what they needed was information about prevention. So many things affect your health, and many health problems can be prevented if you simply learn what you are doing that harms your health as well as what you can do to enhance it.

Cholesterol and fats have been subjects of much interest lately in the news. You may have read recently that it is not cholesterol but sugar that damages your arteries. Some news articles you may read say it is now safe to eat fats. But medical research has affirmed that over half of deaths are caused by disease in the arteries of the heart and the brain that results in heart attacks and strokes. So what information should a person rely on concerning cholesterol and fats?

Since the aging process is determined by the health of your arteries, it is important for you to know the truth about cholesterol and fats and the effect each has on blood vessels. There are ways to prevent processes that damage your arteries, and knowing what you should be doing is the key to good health.

That is why I would like to become your personal "book doctor." There is medical information you need to know. The more you understand your health from a medical perspective, the easier it will be for you to develop lifestyles that will improve your health. I realize you have a physician who knows your medical history and physical condition. I do not want to change one thing they have told you to do or not to do. If you ever have a question concerning your health or medication, I refer you to your doctor, who knows your specific conditions.

However, personal physicians rarely have the time to go into the details of your health as thoroughly as you are going to read about in this book. You may have recently been prescribed a statin drug to lower your cholesterol and told you need to lose weight and exercise. You were probably given a pamphlet or instruction sheet explaining the side effects you may encounter from the medicine. Your doctor may have explained the basic concept of what is going on in your body. Those instructions are good building blocks. But you also need information that will help you prevent problems that will likely occur unless you make changes. That is why I wrote this book.

This book provides a review of the medical literature in terms you can understand. You will learn what your cholesterol numbers mean and why they are so important to your health. After reading this book, you will never have to ask yourself whether you should eat certain fats or not. You will learn the bad fats to avoid and the good fats to eat plenty of.

Your eating habits will change, not because I or your doctor or someone else tells you to avoid particular foods but because you will know what each bite of certain foods can do to your arteries and how the damage those foods can cause leads to heart attacks and strokes. You will look at some foods you now enjoy with a completely different attitude because you will have learned what they are doing to you and how they determine your future. The more you learn medically, the more you will want to not eat the bad and to eat the good.

You will develop a personal exercise program that fits your condition. You will learn about medical research that shows the amazing benefits of doing some form of exercise and the positive impact exercise has on your cholesterol levels. You may not start out enjoying your physical activity, but you will do it as regularly as if you were taking a prescription of "exercise medicine" for your health.

Losing weight also improves your cholesterol levels. Only 12 percent of Americans are at their ideal weight. You will learn what the medical literature has to say about the effect being overweight or obese has on your overall health and will learn some essentials to losing excess weight and keeping it off.

What you are about to read is not based on my ideas. It is based on what the medical literature has to say. This book was written by a physician who wants to help as many patients as possible learn how to protect their most prized possession: their health. The information in this book is what you need to know whether you are in your thirties or your eighties. It will explain what is going on in your body from a medical perspective.

I want to become your "book doctor" so we can go over what cholesterol levels mean to your health in more detail than you would get in an office visit. Not only will the advice in this book help you take charge of your cholesterol, but if you diligently apply the suggestions, you can also turn your physiological age clock back quite a few years. Yes, you will add extra years to your life. But even more important, those years will be active, quality years—beginning today.

I look forward to many follow-up office visits with you.

Your "book doctor,"
Richard Furman, MD, FACS

Introduction

You may have picked up this book because you just saw your doctor, and they told you your cholesterol is high. Maybe a friend just had a heart attack, and you have taken an interest in your health. This book will help you understand cholesterol and its impact on your body. It will help you understand that not all fat is bad. Bad fats and good fats affect your cholesterol differently. And as an added benefit, everything you do to improve your cholesterol numbers will make an impact on your overall health and even how long you live.

His name was Bryan. When he was thirty-six years of age, his doctor gave him the bad news that his cholesterol was way too high. What made this news worse was the fact that Bryan's father had had a heart attack when he was fifty-eight years old, and the physician told Bryan he was more prone to have such an attack with his family history. The doctor prescribed a statin drug in an attempt to get Bryan's cholesterol numbers lower.

"What should I do?" he asked me as a friend. "I want to be around for my children, my grandchildren, and my wife."

I looked at the sheet of paper that showed his cholesterol results. Never in my medical career had I seen such high numbers.

"Your total cholesterol is 289. It should be below 200." I looked at his LDL cholesterol and HDL cholesterol as well as the ratio between his HDL and total cholesterol. I knew he did not have any idea what the numbers meant, and this was not the right time for a long discussion on cholesterol levels.

"There are three things you can do that have a significant effect on your cholesterol." I began a simple explanation but was quickly interrupted.

"I'll do them all. Anything you tell me, I'll do. I don't want a heart attack in my fifties."

"Okay, two of the lifestyles that affect your cholesterol you already do. You are at a good weight and you exercise. So that just leaves the foods you eat. What you are eating is the cause of your high cholesterol numbers." I went on to explain that I wanted him to continue exercising and to keep at his weight, which I felt was ideal for him. Then I went over a list of foods he should not eat one bite of for the next two months.

"Then we will get another blood sample and recheck your numbers. Just make sure this plan is okay with your doctor [who was a friend of mine]. Tell him I recommended it for a two-month period, and if your cholesterol isn't down, then you can begin your medication. I assure you he will agree with the plan if you commit to the diet we just went over."

One week later, I was talking to three football coaches, and all three asked me the same question: "What in the world did you say to Bryan the other day about his eating? We can't get him to eat a single French fry."

I smiled. "He's on a special diet. It's one he will probably be on the rest of his life."

His report two months later read: total cholesterol 196. I told him, "Congratulations. You won't have to take your statin, and I think you can get that number even lower. If you keep your bad cholesterol low by avoiding the wrong foods and your good cholesterol high by exercising and maintaining your ideal weight, you will be on the right road to avoiding a heart attack."

"If only my dad had known." That was his first comment. "If only he'd known what to do, I think he was the kind of person who would have done it."

Many patients tell me, "If only I had known." If only they had known what caused them to have a heart attack, they would have lived differently. If only they had known the real danger of smoking, they would not have developed lung cancer. If only they had known red meat was a causative factor of colon cancer, they would have eaten differently. It's the worst phrase a physician can hear.

For more than thirty years, I was a vascular surgeon. I opened arteries that were plugged with plaque and spooned the blockage out. I placed the pieces of plaque in the palm of my hand and felt them with my fingers. I know what plaque is like, and I want you to have the same knowledge I do about what certain foods can do to your body, about the effect exercise has on your health, and about how important it is not to be overweight. With this medical knowledge, getting control of your cholesterol numbers will become easier.

This book is not just my thoughts about how fat and cholesterol affect your body. This material is not something I thought up or a product I am pushing. In this book, I am pulling together the best medical research and summarizing it in an easy-to-understand format. After reading and studying, you will never have to say the dreaded phrase, "If only I had known."

You will know.

The Art of Healthy Arteries

Your arteries play a monumental role in the aging of your body. The flow of blood through your body carries nutrients, oxygen, electrolytes, and essentials that keep your body running like a new engine. That blood is pumped through your system by your heart and is carried by sixty thousand miles of arteries, plus veins. The condition of those arteries determines how well your body is supplied with all it needs to function at 100 percent. As those arteries become damaged, plaque buildup or inflammation can result in a blockage. Both events will cause the blood flow to completely stop or become markedly decreased. The downstream area then becomes starved for oxygen.

Over half of all Americans will die as a result of damage to the arteries of their hearts or brains. Yet this is a preventable process. Don't become one of the statistics. Set aside the time to learn what the medical literature has to say about preventing the aging process. Learn which fats to avoid, which fats are good for you, and the role that the cholesterol in your blood plays in the aging process.

Fat Myths

There is a big misconception in America concerning fats. We have been told for years, "Don't eat fatty foods. Fat causes heart attacks and strokes. Don't eat any fats. They're bad for you."

More recently, people have written articles and even books saying that fat does not cause the problems in our arteries. Fat does not cause heart attacks and strokes and erectile dysfunction. Instead, sugar is the problem. The next time you hear someone say that fat isn't the problem, just realize they are only half right. (A half-truth is still a whole lie.) Not all fats are bad for us, and not all fats are good for our health. It is important to know the difference.

Some types of fat are good for you because they cause an increase in your good "hero" HDL cholesterol. Nuts, fish, and olives are the most common foods that contain the good fat.

Some, but not all, low-fat foods contain additional sugar to improve the taste. That is something to realize, but you must remember that bad fats have a much more pronounced harmful effect on your arteries than sugar. Sugar does affect the health of your arteries, but saturated fat causes the most harm. When you learn to abstain from bad fats, don't replace them with sugar. Replace them with the good fats and the good foods you will learn about in this book: foods such as fruits, vegetables, nuts, peas, whole grains, fish, and olive and canola oil.

Don't replace bad with bad. Replace bad with good.

Prevention versus Symptoms

Someone asked me, "What are the symptoms of high cholesterol?" I needed only one word to answer her. "None." And that is the problem. We have no idea what is going on inside our arteries. Our bad eating habits create a constant increase in the number of LDL cholesterol particles floating around in our blood. For years and years, damage is being done to our arteries without any warning signs, without any symptoms. We continue our routine of gaining a little weight each year, doing less and less exercise, and eating pretty much whatever we want. The damage to our arteries continues until we have a heart attack or a stroke. The same process even leads to erectile dysfunction in men.

You don't have to be a physician to realize you need to do all you can every day to protect the health of your arteries. Eighty-five percent of people over the age of fifty have some significant blockage in the arteries of their heart without experiencing any symptoms.

These individuals haven't had the first pain in their chest. They haven't had any undue shortness of breath. They haven't experienced pain shooting down their left arm. Most individuals over fifty have significant blockages in their arteries, yet they don't know it because there are no red lights that come on to warn them. Two-thirds of the time the first symptom of blockage is a heart attack. There are no bells or whistles before it happens. One day you are going along routinely and suddenly you have a heart attack.

When does this blockage begin? By the age of twelve, 70 percent of children have some fatty deposits in their arteries. Even though the deposits are minute, the beginning of the disease process is there.

So many times the first symptom of high blood cholesterol is a sudden death from a massive heart attack or a massive stroke that leaves you in a wheelchair for the rest of your life—unable to speak. Waiting for symptoms to happen before you change your lifestyles of weight control, food, and exercise is similar to hearing that you have lung cancer and then deciding to quit smoking. It's the right thing to do—but a little late. Don't wait on symptoms. Your health is one of the most prized possessions you will ever have. If your car needs an oil change, you get it to the shop. If your refrigerator quits working properly, you call someone to repair it. Your body is more valuable, so give your health your best care.

Change for Life

The lifestyles of weight control, food, and exercise determine your physiological age. The medical literature shows us how to develop each lifestyle in order to live younger longer.

Recently, I had dinner with a couple, and the wife was telling me about an herb that had made her bad cholesterol go down and her good cholesterol go up. She went on and on about how good it was for her. Her husband sat quietly until she finished and then said that it may have worked for her but it hadn't for him. He had been placed on a statin drug to lower his bad LDL cholesterol. Her response was classic. "You didn't take enough of the supplement. If you had, it would have worked for you."

This conversation illustrates why medical literature is such a good place to find out what really works and what doesn't. Research in medical literature is not based on what works for one wife and not for one husband. It is based on the double-blind-study concept to prove the numbers. "Here's how scientists would test this pill," I explained to them. "They would take two thousand people and give a thousand of them the real herbal pill and the other thousand a placebo that looked identical. Neither group would know whether it had the herb or not. Then after a period of time, blood would be drawn from all the participants to see if the cholesterol level had changed in one group over the other. That is called a double-blind study. There is no guesswork. The pill either works or it doesn't. Such double-blind studies are the basis for approval by the FDA." I hesitated before telling them the next thought. "However, supplements do not go through such a test to see if they work or cause harm."

"Well, I know it worked for me," the wife stated.

"Not for me," the husband replied.

It is simple to do double-blind studies on lifestyles. And these studies have shown that the lifestyles of weight control, food, and exercise are life changing and important. All three of them are also intertwined, one aiding the others when followed and hindering the others when ignored. You need to learn about and follow all three for your best physiological health.

Can't I Just Take a Pill?

Do you know the most prescribed medicine in the world? It is a drug that has a statin in it. Research has shown that such medication helps prevent heart attacks and strokes because it cuts down on the LDL cholesterol particles traveling around in your blood. It is an accepted medical fact that it is important to keep your LDL cholesterol low. Does the fact that almost half of everyone over the age of forty-five is on a medication to lower their cholesterol say something about the most significant health problem we have in America?

What would you say if I told you that the three lifestyles we have mentioned not only will bring your LDL cholesterol down but also will increase your good HDL cholesterol? As you read on, you will learn how all three of the lifestyles affect both LDL and HDL cholesterol.

If someone tells you that your cholesterol level is not important anymore, just remember that the medical community knows that lowering LDL cholesterol has saved thousands of patients from heart attacks and strokes. You can lower your LDL cholesterol in one of two ways: taking a pill or changing your lifestyles. If you are on a cholesterol-lowering drug, listen up. If you read that little paper written in fine print that comes with your prescription, you may be surprised to see there are things you could be doing to avoid having to take the medicine altogether, or at least to take a lower dose, which would mean fewer side effects. That drug information paper says that *if* eating properly, getting to a healthy weight, and exercising do not lower your cholesterol (your LDL cholesterol), then you should take the medicine. I have asked numerous individuals who are on such medication if their physician had them try lifestyle changes (avoiding certain foods, losing weight, and exercising) before prescribing the drug. So far the answer has been no. Most patients are placed on the medication and told that in addition they should work on changing their eating habits and should exercise and lose some weight. But the doctor doesn't have the time to explain the importance of lifestyle changes.

Here is one more factor that will make you think about the importance of changing your lifestyles so you don't have to take medication to lower your cholesterol: side effects. Side effects of any medication are real, but we don't usually pay attention to them until they affect us. Have you ever seen a drug advertisement on television? I don't see how the commercials are effective when they list all the possible dangers associated with the medication. Most people would run from the drug rather than take it if they paid attention to all the possible side effects.

I have a friend who was on a cholesterol-lowering medication, and his leg muscles and joints caused him so much difficulty that he had to use both hands on the handrail when he climbed a flight of stairs. His doctor took him off the statin because he needed to take another medicine that could not be taken with the statin. Within two months, not only was my friend climbing stairs normally, but he was also able to get back on the elliptical machine to exercise.

I asked him, "Did your physician encourage you to develop a diet that would lower your cholesterol, to lose that extra twenty-five pounds you are carrying around, and to set up an exercise plan before he prescribed the cholesterol medicine? Did your doctor explain the difference between good fats and bad fats?"

I remember his blank stare as he answered, "I remember a piece of paper came with the medicine, but I didn't read it. It looked too complicated for me to understand."

I explained that the instruction sheet for cholesterol-lowering medicines begins with a statement that such medicine is indicated *if* eating properly, reaching and maintaining a proper weight, and exercising were not successful in getting the cholesterol to a normal range.

If you are on a cholesterol-lowering drug, you can learn how to get the dose lowered or completely discontinued. There are better ways to control your LDL cholesterol with no side effects. If you start such lifestyle changes, your physician will encourage you wholeheartedly.

A False Sense of Security

Whether trying to lose weight, lower your cholesterol, or avoid a heart attack, don't give yourself a false sense of security. Do you take a baby aspirin daily to prevent a heart attack? Do you know someone who does? Nearly a third of middle-aged Americans regularly take a baby aspirin in hope of preventing a heart attack or a stroke.

A recent article in the medical journal *Archives of Internal Medicine* reported on a study of more than one hundred thousand people who had never had a heart attack or a stroke. They were given either an aspirin or a nonaspirin placebo. Researchers found that the overall risk of dying was the same with both groups. The aspirin takers were 10 percent less likely to have any type of heart event but were 30 percent more likely to have a serious gastrointestinal bleeding event, a side effect of frequent aspirin use.

The report concluded that for people without a previous heart attack or stroke, the regular use of aspirin may be more harmful than it is beneficial. If you are taking an aspirin without being directed to do so by your doctor, ask your physician if you should be taking it. Don't use it as a false sense of security. There are many things you can do that have a much more profound effect on preventing a heart attack.

If you are trying to take something to prevent a clot from forming, you should also be making lifestyle changes. If you are not living a heart- and artery-friendly lifestyle and are only taking an aspirin, you are going bear hunting with a switch.

It is much more important to know the difference between good fats and bad. It is much more important to give up the bad fats and replace them with the good. It is good that people who take a baby aspirin daily are interested in their health. Much more significant is that they make the commitment to develop healthy lifestyles that protect them. The worse type of trick you can play on yourself is to eat a dinner high in saturated fat and then go home and take an aspirin to "protect" yourself from a heart attack. Focus on preventing the *cause* of a blood clot forming in a heart artery rather than concentrating on what may help after such a clot forms.

Develop the lifestyles of weight control, proper eating, and exercise to keep your LDL down and to get your HDL up. If your doctor recommends that you take an aspirin, by all means take it while you are making the big three lifestyle changes.

I was eating dinner with some friends who told me an interesting story about a friend of theirs who took an aspirin to prevent a heart attack. He was in his late fifties and was found dead in his car on the side of the road. His father was in a rest home, and he was on his way to visit him. He had complained of some sort of strange feeling in his chest earlier in the day, but he didn't think it was significant. A few hours later, someone stopped to see why a driver was just sitting in a car on the side of the road. He was not breathing. His heart had stopped. There was nothing that could be done. Beside him on the seat was a new bottle of aspirin. It had been opened. But the aspirin couldn't save him. Don't fool the person in the mirror.

Years ago, I made some dramatic changes in my life after I reviewed the medical literature. Knowing what the medical literature said motivated me to commit to not eating certain foods, exercising regularly, and sustaining an ideal weight. I want you to have a similar experience as you read this book.

▶ **Action Steps**

1. Recruit an accountability partner or organize a support group to help you develop a plan. Determine how often you will communicate about your progress. Develop your goals together.

2. Buy two or three types of fat-free salad dressing to replace your current dressings at home.

3. Eat nothing fried for the next week.

PART 1

TAKING CHARGE

1. Cholesterol Matters

We have a problem. Most people do not know what is going on in their bodies. The damage happens quietly, and most people have no idea that what they are doing is causing the damage.

Your overall health is determined in large part by the health of your arteries. Your heart is the pump, and your arteries are the conduit responsible for carrying every particle necessary to keep your body functioning properly. If you learn nothing else concerning your anatomy related to your health, take note of the importance of the health of your arteries. Your arteries are the pipeline for the nutrients that are essential to every cell in your body. If that pipeline is partially plugged, you are setting yourself up for problems, especially in your heart and brain. Keep the health of your arteries at the forefront of your thinking as you continue reading this book.

Picture in your mind small particles floating around in your blood. Some of these particles are good; some are bad. The bad particles work their way through the lining of an artery and get stuck in the wall itself. This causes a reaction in which cells and fluids mix in an attempt to get rid of the foreign particle that has invaded the wall of the artery. Over time, this reaction can lead to either a rupture or plaque buildup in the affected artery. This is a silent process. It doesn't cause you pain. It doesn't give you a headache or make your chest hurt. It works quietly while you order extra cheese on your hamburger and ask for extra cream sauce on your steak.

The health of our arteries is one of the greatest health problems in America and one that results in over half of our deaths every year. We all need to learn and remind ourselves what happens in our bodies as we go about our daily lives. We need to know what the numbers represent when the doctor hands us our cholesterol reports. We need to know that blood cholesterol is completely different from dietary cholesterol. One is in blood, and the other is in food. The cholesterol in our blood affects our arteries directly. The cholesterol in certain foods can cause our blood cholesterol to become elevated. You are going to learn which foods have the most profound effect on your blood cholesterol. I encourage you to avoid as many of the foods that elevate your blood cholesterol as possible.

Most people do not realize that not all cholesterol is bad. Just as there is good fat, there is also good cholesterol. You are about to learn the difference as a physician understands it, and you won't have to go to medical school to find out.

Cholesterol: More Than Just a Number

Cholesterol is a fatty substance in the outer layer of every cell in your body that maintains each cell's membrane. It is involved in the production of sex hormones as well as hormones released by your adrenal glands. It insulates nerve fibers. It is significant in the metabolizing of certain vitamins, including A, D, and E. It is essential to your body. Cholesterol is carried through the bloodstream combined with a protein. The structure of the cholesterol with the protein is a molecule called a lipoprotein. There are two main types of lipoproteins. They appear on your lab report as Low Density Lipoprotein and High Density Lipoprotein, or LDL and HDL. Here is an easy way to remember them: LDL is "lethal," and HDL is a "hero." You want your lethal number to be as low as possible and your hero number to be as high as possible.

Your cholesterol numbers are to your body what warning lights are to your car. If you are like many people, you don't know your numbers, or if you know them, you don't realize the significance of abnormal numbers. If you don't know your cholesterol numbers, get a test done today to find out what they are. You have to notice a warning light before you can take action.

By the Numbers

Let's look at what doctors mean when they talk about cholesterol numbers. There are three important numbers: the total cholesterol, the LDL cholesterol, and the HDL cholesterol.

When your doctor tells you your cholesterol is too high, they are usually talking about your total cholesterol number. But most patients don't realize that the total cholesterol is the sum of their bad LDL cholesterol and their good HDL cholesterol. There are some additional cholesterol particles within that total number, but they are fairly insignificant to understanding what is going on.

When your physician says your cholesterol is too high, they actually means your LDL cholesterol is too high. This is because your total cholesterol number is made up mostly of your lethal LDL cholesterol, and if it is high, your total number is high.

If you are told you must get your cholesterol down, your doctor means you should get your LDL cholesterol down. When your physician says to start on a cholesterol-lowering medication, what they should say is that they are going to start you on an LDL cholesterol–lowering medication. Your doctor should then explain that the primary cause of high LDL cholesterol is eating foods that contain the bad fats.

Lethal LDL Cholesterol

Let me give you an illustration of how LDL cholesterol affects your arteries.

Picture what happens when a splinter gets stuck in your finger. The area of the penetration becomes a battleground. The body responds initially by pouring fluid into the space around the splinter. The fluid contains numerous specialized cells that are expert at fighting the foreign body. One of two things then happens. The area either ruptures and drains, or it heals with cells that cause thick scar tissue.

The same process happens when an LDL cholesterol particle gets stuck in the wall of one of your arteries. That LDL particle is like the splinter. The LDL splinter causes your body to send out the inflammatory army to that battleground in the wall of the invaded artery. Again, one of two things happens. The area swells with inflammation that ruptures into the artery, which results in immediate clot formation and blockage of that artery, like a straw plugging up, or the battle ensues until fibroblast cells surround the enemy LDL particle and wall it off, forming a scar, which is known as plaque.

The LDL cholesterol splinters do not pick and choose which arterial wall they are going to get into, but the ones we hear about the most are the ones that cause the most dramatic symptoms and damage. These are the arteries in the heart and the brain. Heart attacks and strokes are the result.

The damage takes years to accumulate and often happens numerous times at the same places, usually where there is turbulence in the blood flow, such as where an artery divides or where a smaller artery branches off from a larger one. If there is repeated healing and scarring, plaque builds up until it finally gets large enough to cause a complete blockage of the artery.

When a splinter gets in your finger, you make sure you don't stick your finger into the briar patch again. But the problem with cholesterol is that when the LDL splinters get in the wall of an artery, no pain is involved. You don't realize it is happening over and over. There is no pain to warn you. You have to learn from medical research.

Hero HDL Cholesterol

The component that is often skipped when considering cholesterol numbers is that you should do everything possible to get your HDL cholesterol higher in addition to getting your LDL cholesterol down.

The cholesterol that usually gets left out of the discussion is the good, hero HDL cholesterol. However, the HDL number is as important as the LDL number in understanding how damage to your arteries comes about and what can be done to protect them. In fact, the American Heart Association lists a significantly low HDL as a cause of heart disease. It is as bad as hypertension or obesity when it comes to causing a heart attack. Therefore, physicians should educate their patients on what can be done to raise HDL even though there is no medication they can prescribe for it.

HDL cholesterol is of equal significance to LDL cholesterol because HDL cholesterol combats LDL cholesterol, which is the culprit causing problems in the heart arteries, brain arteries, or any other artery in your body. If your HDL is below 40, you are in a separate medical category of cardiac danger. Here is the way to picture how HDL particles work.

Think of HDL particles as patrol cars that cruise through your blood looking for lethal LDL cholesterol splinters. An HDL particle pulls up by an arterial wall that has several LDL splinters in it, puts them into the patrol car, and takes them to jail—the liver—which disposes of them. Then the HDL patrol car goes back to pick up more LDL splinters to take them to the liver. The more of these patrol cars you have, the better. As a matter of fact, for every point increase in HDL, there is a 2 to 3 percent decrease in your chance of having a heart attack.

There is no medication to increase your HDL. The two lifestyles that play the biggest role in controlling your HDL cholesterol are your weight and how much you exercise. The more you weigh, the lower your HDL is going to be. As you lose excess weight, your HDL will increase. Exercise does the same thing; the more intense your exercise, the higher your HDL cholesterol will get.

The Importance of the Ratio of Total Cholesterol to HDL Cholesterol

The more HDL patrol cars you have and the fewer LDL splinters you have, the better. That means you need to do all you can to avoid the foods that cause your LDL to increase. At the same time, you need to do all you can to increase the number of HDL particles in your arsenal of battleground equipment. The two biggest weapons are exercise and weight loss. The cholesterol number that is often the least explained is the ratio of total cholesterol to HDL cholesterol. If you were to divide your total cholesterol number by your HDL cholesterol number, the more HDL cholesterol you have, the lower that ratio would be. This shows the importance of having as much HDL as possible to fight the battle and as few LDL enemies as possible to fight against.

Let's say that in your total cholesterol number there is one unit of HDL and four units of LDL. If you add them together, you would have five units for your total cholesterol. If you divide your total cholesterol by your HDL, you would get a ratio of 5.0. Now let's say you have two units of HDL and four units of LDL, giving a total of six units. If you divide your total cholesterol of six by your HDL of two, your ratio falls to 3.0. You want your ratio to be below 3.5. Even if your LDL stays the same, you can drop your ratio by raising your HDL.

The importance of the ratio of total cholesterol to HDL makes you realize the significance of your HDL cholesterol. Remember that statin drugs affect only the LDL cholesterol part of the picture. If you avoid foods that contribute to your LDL number while at the same time losing weight and exercising, which increases your HDL number, you will improve your ratio. There is so much more you can do to protect your arteries than take a pill to help lower your LDL cholesterol. Don't focus on one aspect of the battle. Fight the full fight.

Look at the whole picture of what is happening and go after quality health.

No medication can protect you as much as you can protect yourself by taking proper care of your body. Statins have been shown to prevent many heart attacks by lowering a person's LDL cholesterol. If your doctor has you on such a medication, by all means take it, but be sure to talk to your physician about your commitment to make lifestyle changes that should make it possible for you to decrease or even eliminate the medicine. Your physician will keep a record of your HDL to total cholesterol ratio. Aim high and shoot for a ratio below 3.5.

Good Choices and Bad Choices

If you don't know which foods are bad, you will continue to choose the kinds of foods that result in damage that causes over half of the deaths in America. Once you know good and bad choices and the result of each, your eating lifestyle will change.

Let me give you an example. I took a flight from Cusco, Peru, to Lima, Peru, and had a two-and-a-half-hour layover. The fellow I was traveling with had credentials to get us into the airline lounge. We went to the nicest flight lounge I had ever seen. There was a room designated as a quiet zone with large padded lounge chairs and dimmed lighting. (Most of the people in the room were asleep, and I wondered if any would miss their plane.) The food was markedly different from that of other lounges I had visited. There was a long table with a machine in the middle that produced fresh-squeezed orange juice. The attendant placed whole oranges into the top, and you could watch them being sliced in two and carried to a rounded grinder that produced juice, which fell to the bottom of the see-through box. It was entertaining to watch.

To the right of the orange juice machine were the healthy foods: a multitude of different nuts, bowls of olives, and fruits.

To the left were fried bananas, small sandwiches of processed meat mixed with some type of mayonnaise, chocolates of all shapes, at least three types of cakes with creamy icing, and some type of fried chips I didn't recognize.

If the people in charge of the food knew about bad fats and good fats, they could not have done a better job of showing the public which foods they should eat and which they should avoid.

This food selection was going to be my dinner, because in a couple of hours I was going to board an overnight flight back to the United States. I planned to sleep the full seven hours rather than spend the first two hours waiting for dinner to be served on the aircraft.

Let me tell you what I ate because I knew which foods cause the lethal LDL to increase and which foods cause the hero HDL to increase. Three mainstay food types ran through my mind: fish, nuts, and olives or olive oil (or canola oil). These foods contain the good fats—the healthy monounsaturated fat and the good omega-3s. I didn't see any fish, but I saw a large selection of nuts and olives as well as an orange and a banana. I filled my plate and took a seat.

I wondered what my friend would get. He didn't understand that his eating habits were causing disease to his arteries. He got every fried item they had. He quickly ate several sandwiches with the processed meat hidden in mayonnaise globs and went back for seconds. He even had a third helping of whatever the little fried fingerlings were. Then he went back for the chocolates.

Why? I kept asking myself. Why do individuals not pay attention to what medical research shows us about how to keep our bodies at peak performance? That is my goal in this book: to condense the best medical research for you in easy-to-understand terms, to tell you what things you can control that will allow you to decide how you want to live. Then it is up to you to choose. I am hoping you will commit to quality choices for life.

Your Numbers Do Matter

In my study hangs a plaque a friend gave me that reads, "If you are going to be stupid, you've got to be tough." I will admit I did some stupid things that inspired my friend to give me the plaque, but I encourage you to seek wisdom, not be tough, when it comes to protecting your most valuable possession—your health.

Money can't buy extra years for your life. The Bible states that money can't keep us from the grave. All must die someday. But the following information from the medical literature proves that though we can't avoid the grave, we can add years to our lives and improve the quality of the years we have.

The *Journal of the American Medical Association* reported a study on the life expectancy of men who had favorable total cholesterol levels compared to men of the same age who had unfavorable total cholesterol levels. The results astounded me, and I think they will astound you too. The men who had the favorable total cholesterol levels had a life expectancy that was 3.8 to 8.7 years longer than that of those with the unfavorable total cholesterol levels. There was a continuous, proportional relationship between total cholesterol and life expectancy. The men who took their eating habits the most seriously had the 8.7-year increase.

These figures alone give you a huge insight into the importance of controlling what you are doing to your body. High total cholesterol spells danger because the total cholesterol number consists mostly of the lethal LDL cholesterol. So the next time you order a steak with a creamy cheese sauce, butter on your baked potato, and fried green tomatoes as your vegetable, realize how expensive that meal is, and I am not talking dollars. Years of your life are a lot to pay just because you didn't know what you were buying.

Here are several more statistics that will motivate you to do something to increase the quality of your life. The facts show that you have over a 50 percent chance of dying from disease in your arteries—a heart attack or a stroke. Look yourself in the mirror and repeat that number. Unless you do something to protect your health, the odds are against you. Only 7.6 percent of people who suffer a complete cardiac arrest outside of a hospital setting survive long enough to be discharged. One-half of individuals who die from cardiac arrest are under the age of sixty-five. Just because you are not in your eighties doesn't mean you don't need to take care of your arteries. And a most significant statistic: people with high cholesterol have about *twice* the risk of heart disease as individuals with lower levels.

As we continue this journey, I believe you will begin to think differently about eating certain bad foods. You will visualize in your mind exactly what a particular item is going to do to you. I guarantee you will have less and less desire for it the more you are reminded what it is doing to your body. There are two types of people. Type one will hear the statistics and do something with the information. Type two will hear the numbers and continue with life as usual. Which are you?

"If only I had known." Now you know.

▶ Action Steps

1. Get your blood cholesterol checked today.

2. Record your numbers and compare them with the healthy range to see where you fit. Circle any numbers that fall outside the healthy range—these are your warning signs.

    _____: total cholesterol (healthy range below 200)

    _____: LDL cholesterol (healthy range below 100)

    _____: HDL cholesterol (healthy range above 40 if male, above 50 if female)

    _____: total cholesterol/HDL ratio (healthy range below 3.5)

3. If you know anyone on a statin, ask them to let you see the prescription insert that came with the medicine. Read the side effects.

4. Eat three fruits with your breakfast for the next week.

2. Three Lifestyles That Will Change Your Life

Desire takes place in the mind and requires no action. You desire to lose weight, but when you are offered a sundae or a chocolate candy bar, you cave. After indulging to the very last bite, you realize your desire to lose weight was assaulted and the momentary pleasure was fulfilled. Then you wish you hadn't eaten it. You desired to lose weight, but when you were confronted with a choice, your desire was not strong enough to win the battle. The problem with having only a desire is that desire is of the mind and requires no action.

Commitment, on the other hand, speaks of duty, obligation, or a heavy responsibility. You have thought about something, made a decision, and turned that decision of your mind into a commitment. Commitment demands action.

Once you are committed to a healthier life, the next step is changing your "want to's." You will change from "I love cheese and fried foods and red meat" to "I know what certain foods do to my cholesterol level and my health." I want to be active until I die. I want to be able to continue playing tennis. I want to be able to travel with my spouse. I want to be able to continue doing the things I am now doing. Commitment will change what you want to eat. Commitment will make you want to exercise to improve the strength of your heart, which pumps nutrition throughout your body. You will want to get to an ideal weight so you can be more active, improve your cholesterol numbers, and even help prevent common types of cancer. You will look at lifestyle changes as positive actions rather than something you have to give up. I encourage you to commit to changing your negative lifestyles into positive ones to create the physiologically youngest body you can achieve.

"How do you turn a desire into a commitment?" you ask.

Everybody loves secrets. I want to introduce you to a secret of self-control that I have shared with patients over the years. It will allow you to be successful in taking charge of your weight, your eating habits, and your arterial blockages. This one factor will help free you from snacking. It will help you walk away from that piece of chocolate. It will help you order salad with succulent grilled chicken instead of fried chicken and French fries. It is the most important self-control tool I know. It is called the ten-minute factor. This dynamic component of reasoning doesn't suggest what you can do— it demands you do it (at least for a period of ten minutes). How hard can that be?

We consume many foods because we are addicted to them. To beat a food addiction, you have to defeat the desire for that food. You can't do this through moderation. Deciding to eat a certain type of food only once a week is like a smoker saying they will smoke only on Saturdays. No, you have to abstain. And it takes about sixty days for the desire for a particular food to weaken. The desire will become less and less until the time comes when you couldn't care less if you added cheese to your sandwich or if you ate that steak or bowl of ice cream.

The Ten-Minute Factor

The ten-minute factor works like this: when you have a desire for a food you shouldn't eat, you tell yourself you are not going to eat it for ten minutes. Then you drink a glass of a noncaloric beverage instead of eating the food. Next, you do something active. You take a walk, talk with someone on the phone, plan an activity. If the same urge hits you an hour later, you repeat the ten-minute factor.

I got this idea from a man I met in Alaska years ago. It worked for him, and it works for me and many of my patients. This man had a smoking problem, a drinking problem, and a drug problem. He told me that he was an expert on addiction because he had three addictions at the same time. Yet he overcame them all by practicing the ten-minute factor.

He realized he could control an addiction for about ten minutes. "I learned that if I could avoid the craving at that time and begin doing something else, I could turn that ten minutes into hours of avoidance." I will never forget the look on his face when he told me that. He had complete confidence in what he was telling me. He pointed out that he didn't tell himself he was never going to smoke another cigarette, just that he was not going to smoke for the next ten minutes. Then he would get busy doing something else, and the desire would weaken.

41

I have shared this principle with patients who were trying to lose weight or stop smoking. I remember encouraging a patient who smoked with the ten-minute factor. I had removed a mass from his left lung that was benign. We were both happy with the results, but I informed him that if he didn't quit smoking two packs a day, eventually he would develop a malignant tumor in his lung. I asked him if he were standing in the middle of the road in front of my office and a tractor trailer truck was coming down the hill right toward him if he would get out of the road so it wouldn't hit him. He laughed and said, "Of course I would." I explained that lung cancer was that truck coming right at him, and he needed to quit smoking that day or he was destined to get run over. I explained the ten-minute factor to him, and he left my office. For some reason, I didn't expect him to quit smoking. I didn't think he had the commitment or even the desire to quit. I didn't see him again for a long time.

Then one day my office nurse said there was a man who wanted to see me. "In the hallway is okay with him. He doesn't have an appointment."

I was busy but said, "Go get him. I'll see him right now."

He was in his work clothes and a ball cap. He had the biggest smile of any patient that day. He stuck his hand out to shake mine. "It's been a year today," he said. "I just wanted to let you know it worked." He smiled even bigger as he explained, "When I left your office, I laid my pack of cigarettes on the dash of my truck. Every time I wanted one, I just told myself that I wasn't going to smoke for the next ten minutes. Every time I wanted one, I put it off and got to doing something else. It's been one year today, and I just wanted you to know." As he turned to walk away, I recalled his earlier struggle and congratulated him. He had learned the art of the ten-minute factor.

The ten-minute factor is a great tool for making food choices as well. We will go into more detail later on how to apply it to weight control, so don't forget its importance. It is not a secret anymore.

Your Goal for Life

Improving your cholesterol is one part of a much bigger picture. How do you want to live out the rest of your life? How do you want to live out this next year? Next week? And probably the most important question is, How do you want to live out the rest of today?

Have you ever written a goal on a sticky note and put it on your mirror? A goal is everything. The higher your goal, the more success you will achieve. A goal can be the difference between failing or not failing to take proper care of your most prized possession: your health. Setting a goal is essential to succeeding at losing excess weight, maintaining an exercise program, or eating certain foods. Without a goal, you can't make something happen. You can memorize every weight-loss secret, but you won't lose weight—unless you have a goal.

Researchers at the Rush University Medical Center in Chicago interviewed more than twelve hundred elderly adults and found something interesting concerning setting goals. Researchers aren't certain why, but the study found that over the next five years, the individuals who had goals were about half as likely to die as those who didn't have definite plans for the future. I encourage you to set lifestyle goals and write them down. Ninety-three percent of people never set goals. Be part of the 7 percent who do and see how goals help you improve your health.

Before I set my lifestyle goals, I read articles in credible medical journals. The more I read, the more I realized that the health of our arteries determines our aging process. It became evident that we can turn back physiological age quite a few years if we take control of three lifestyles. Based on my research, I made the following goals: (1) I will eat the proper foods and eliminate the ones that cause damage to my arteries; (2) I will exercise daily; and (3) I will get to and maintain my ideal weight.

After a few years, I wondered if sticking to these health goals was paying off. I felt great, but I didn't have any medical proof that my lifestyle changes were working. Let me tell you the story of the day I got the proof that eating properly, exercising, and sustaining an ideal weight were making a difference in my health.

A friend who is eleven years younger than me invited me to go with him to the Cooper Clinic in Dallas to have a complete medical workup. Doctors would perform laboratory blood tests, an EKG, a stress test, a proctoscopy colon exam, arterial studies, and other tests that would determine the physical shape of our bodies.

At the end of the day, they sat us down and reviewed their findings. The primary doctor invited me to sit in a soft leather chair as he began. "I want to give you our findings for the day. From a cardiac standpoint, you are . . ." He paused before smiling. "Now, listen to this next word." He smiled again. "*Above* the ninety-ninth percentile." He nodded his head a few times. "I just wanted you to know that whatever you are doing with your exercise and weight control, continue doing it."

He went through my blood tests, pointing out that my cholesterol numbers were great. He told me my colon was clear of any polyps or diverticula. On and on he went, making me realize that all the medical literature I had read and applied was paying off.

Then he made a defining statement that made me realize the lifestyle changes I had made were worth it. He ended the review by stating, "The best part of the report is that physiologically you are one year younger than your friend, who is eleven years younger than you chronologically."

I tell you this story to encourage you to do all you can to get as physiologically young as possible. It is worth setting the proper lifestyle goals to follow the rest of your life to get to and remain seven to twelve years younger physiologically than you are chronologically.

From time to time, that same friend reminds me that I am getting older. When we ride our motorcycles to Alaska from North Carolina, he comments that I may not have too many more opportunities to take such rides because I am getting older. I then remind him that I am younger than he is physiologically and that he is the one he ought to be concerned about.

Because of that trip to the clinic, I know the medical literature I have read is true and trustworthy. I know it works from a medical standpoint. I know it is not just my take on how to develop a healthier life. The three lifestyles put into practice what the medical literature has to say about how our bodies work and what we can do to make them work at peak performance.

Keep your engine functioning at the ninety-ninth percentile compared to everyone else your age—and encourage your friends and family to do the same.

Three Lifestyles You Can Control

You can't control the color of your eyes or your blood type or your genes. But there are three distinct lifestyles you can regulate: weight control, food, and exercise. Not only do you have control over them, but you are also constantly encouraging them to be what they are whether you realize it or not.

The first lifestyle over which you have control is your weight. Everyone has an ideal weight. Sadly, two-thirds of all Americans are either overweight or obese. Only 12 percent are at their ideal weight, and only 2 to 20 percent of people who lose weight are able to sustain that weight loss. We will go over a formula later based on your gender and height that will give you a good goal for your ideal weight.

The second lifestyle involves food. You control the foods you eat and those you don't eat. In this book, you will learn the difference between good fats and bad fats and the effect blood cholesterol has on your arteries. Based on medical research, this book will answer questions such as, What is the proof that certain bad fats do harm? Are there good fats I should be eating? How do they help rather than cause damage?

You have probably read many mixed reports about cholesterol and find them confusing. Can cholesterol be explained in such a way that you can understand the difference between the *blood cholesterol* report you get from your doctor and the *dietary cholesterol* found in foods such as egg yolk? Are these completely different cholesterols? If so, why are they used interchangeably in so many articles? These are questions I want to answer so you will see the benefits of changing your food lifestyle.

The third lifestyle is exercise. Most people see exercise as a way to burn calories, but the caloric benefits of exercise are minute compared to some other amazing benefits.

Over half of Americans are sedentary; they sit all evening and watch television. They do no exercise at all. The medical literature reveals that if you can't walk a quarter of a mile in five minutes, you are thirty times more likely to die within the next three years than someone who can walk that quarter mile in five minutes.

I am not saying you will die in three years if you don't exercise at all. But I am saying that people who exercise do a better job taking care of their bodies than people who are sedentary. People who exercise also tend to eat better and weigh less. Similar articles point out that jogging increases life expectancy by an average of six years. I am not saying that everyone should be able to run three eight-minute miles six days a week, but I am saying that going on a brisk walk for thirty minutes a day six days a week is a thousand times more beneficial than sitting on the couch and doing nothing.

Exercise has another wonderful side effect. Exercise lets your mind know you are committed to getting younger physiologically. You can't fool yourself. If you exercise, your mind gets it—you are committed. If you don't exercise, your chance of losing weight is slim (no pun intended).

There are many forms of exercise. At first, you may have to tell yourself that even if you don't like getting on the treadmill every day, you are going to treat it as you do taking medicine. You wouldn't skip taking a medicine as prescribed. Treadmill or pill? That is the question, and I encourage you to get started on prevention rather than being treated with a pill for the rest of your life.

Here is another benefit of exercise. A pill, such as a statin, does nothing to strengthen your heart muscle. Only exercise can do that. If I were to take you to anatomy class in medical school, you could see several hearts. If the professor held up a heart from someone who had exercised a lot, you would notice the thickness of the muscle. You would see muscle that measured about an inch from wall to wall. If the professor showed you one from a couch potato, a person who was completely sedentary, who didn't exercise at all, you would see a heart muscle only about a quarter inch in thickness or less.

The stronger the muscle is, the less effort it takes to pump an equivalent amount of blood throughout the body in comparison to the thin, weaker muscle. The stronger the heart muscle is, the less oxygen it requires to do its work.

Exercise is the key to strengthening the muscle in your heart. I encourage you to develop the strongest heart you can. That is the one organ your body depends on the most. It is the engine that drives your body. Protect it now so you won't have problems later on. Don't wait for symptoms. From now on, think prevention first.

The Choice Is Yours

Place your decisions on a scale and weigh them. Place "this food will cause disease of my arteries" on one side of the scale and place "this food will keep my arteries safe" on the other. Couch potato on one side of the scale versus exercise on the other. Snacks and being overweight on one side and ideal weight on the other.

Be realistic with yourself. If you are going to make choices, at least place them on a scale and admit to yourself where your choices will lead. If you walk through an office, most of the people who are overweight have food on their desks or in a drawer. If you have junk food in your desk, see it as food on the bad side of the scale and throw it away. Acknowledge what the scale is telling you and take action. The same goes for the wrong foods in your kitchen at home. Throw them away. Empty the bad side of the scale, which represents the wrong side of the three lifestyles.

Think of your cholesterol numbers as you would the warning lights on your car. If your numbers are high, take action to change them to get your heart and arteries running at peak performance.

Now that you have learned a way to control your desires, you have completed the first step in learning how to take charge of your cholesterol numbers and, more than that, to live younger for a longer period of time. Gaining some basic medical knowledge of what goes on in your body as well as in your mind will prove invaluable as you move forward and apply the ten-minute factor.

When I was in med school, every night after dinner I would study my notes until midnight. I am not suggesting you go back over this information on cholesterol until 12 a.m., but I do recommend you take some time to review what we have been saying about total cholesterol, LDL cholesterol, and HDL cholesterol so that whenever you are going to eat a certain food that will cause your LDL to increase, you will choose not to take a bite. And you will make wise choices about exercising and getting to an ideal weight. You want to make a good grade when it comes to choices that will determine your physiological age.

▷ Action Steps

1. Write down three options for activities you can do when you apply the ten-minute factor to beat your food cravings.
2. Practice the ten-minute factor to completely eliminate snacks for the next seven days.
3. The next time you fill up your car with gasoline, go into the convenience store, pick up a Snickers bar, and read how much saturated fat it contains. Place it back on the shelf and do the same with a package of Oreo cookies.

PART 2

LIFESTYLE 1:

WEIGHT CONTROL

3. Losing Weight and Keeping It Off

The majority of overweight people who want to lose weight are concerned about one thing: appearance. They want to look better. But appearance is unimportant compared to the damage you do to your body if you remain overweight.

Your risk for becoming diabetic increases tremendously.

Your risk for becoming hypertensive increases significantly.

Being overweight is a significant cause of breast cancer.

Being overweight is one of the known causes of colon cancer.

Medical studies show a direct correlation between body weight and mortality.

There is a direct correlation between being overweight and heart disease.

"But my problem is cholesterol. Why should weight matter to me?"

I'm glad you asked.

The correlation between weight and cholesterol is one of the most important lessons about losing weight. Remember that hero HDL cholesterol particles are the patrol cars, and you want as many HDL particles as possible traveling through your bloodstream. Losing weight increases your HDL cholesterol particles. And remember that for every point your HDL increases, your chance of developing heart disease or having a heart attack decreases by 2 to 3 percent. The opposite side of that coin is that obesity can raise LDL cholesterol by as much as 50 percent and lower HDL cholesterol by 20 to 30 percent.

You may not classify yourself as obese, but remember we are talking degrees. Even being at the lower end of the overweight or obese scale affects your HDL and LDL to some degree.

Only 2 to 20 percent of those who lose weight actually keep it off. Think of that. Eighty to 98 percent of those who lose weight regain it and frequently add additional pounds. This is staggering! You "lose" the battle in the end, because regained pounds are usually created by foods that cause your LDL cholesterol to increase, putting more LDL splinters into the walls of your arteries.

Two-thirds of people in our nation are either overweight or obese. That means only one-third of Americans are of normal weight by Body Mass Index (BMI) standards. You will learn about BMI later, but just because you are in the normal range does not mean you are at your ideal weight. In actuality, only 12 percent of Americans are at their ideal weight. Do you recall that having a high LDL cholesterol versus having a low LDL cholesterol could rob you of 8.7 years of your life expectancy? Excess weight is also a costly error. Being overweight takes six years off your life expectancy. Nothing good happens as a result of being overweight.

Why Diets Don't Work

Let me tell you about the head of a large organization. We will call him Jim. He travels a lot. As someone who has traveled a good bit myself, I know it is difficult to maintain good eating habits while on the road. This is the case with Jim. He will drop the extra pounds, but before long his clothes—and the scale—reflect that he has invited the unwelcome weight right back into his life.

Jim dresses nicely, but soon his abdomen pushes tightly against his belt, and he has to let it out a notch. Then the shirttails that were once neatly tucked into the waist of his pants begin to peek out over his belt. At that point, Jim goes back on his routine diet, which consists of nothing but protein: usually pork or steak and sometimes chicken. He has discipline because he eats no bread—just meat! It isn't long before the weight begins to come off. He begins to look more trim, and his clothes begin to fit a little better. After two or three months, Jim is back to his normal weight.

One could argue that his plan works, except that in the process his purely protein diet damages his arteries, and he is on a constant cycle of losing and regaining pounds around his waistline. What Jim doesn't realize is that the protein diet he eats to lose weight is composed of some of the worst foods he could eat. He doesn't realize that the red meat and pork are full of saturated fat, which causes an increase in the number of LDL splinters that get into the walls of his arteries, especially those in his heart and brain. There is a reason why his diet doesn't work and never will.

Next consider John, a physician. He works long and stressful hours and is certainly not a chef. Probably 95 percent of his meals come from restaurants and fast-food establishments. He tries to stay in shape. He jogs at least five days a week and even has some weights in his den to keep his muscles toned. He is proud that he works on one lifestyle: exercise. But the other two lifestyles, the foods he eats and his weight control, are left by the wayside. He has the desire to improve them, but he is so busy with his medical practice that he never gets around to losing weight or eating properly.

Then one evening a television ad catches his attention. Trim and fit men and women who look like movie stars are shown standing next to pictures taken when they weren't so trim and fit. In fact, they all had been thirty to fifty pounds heavier just one year ago. A man who had played professional football stands in front of the camera. John can see his abs as clearly as if each muscle had been outlined with a marker. One of the women smiles beautifully as she stands beside her before picture. They talk as if losing the weight was not difficult at all. They are convincing. "If I can do it, so can you." All you have to do is order the diet plan. You don't have to cook. You don't have to do anything but use an oven or a microwave or add a little water. The ad shows pictures of the food you will receive in the mail. It looks so appetizing and even includes desserts. Actually, the desserts look like the best part of the deal. You get to eat anything you like or want. To John, the price isn't all that bad either. Especially since he eats out almost every meal anyway.

You know where this is leading, don't you? John does exactly what you are thinking. He signs up for the plan. And it works. In a month's time, he loses weight. As the months go on, he loses more and more. Everyone tells him how good he looks and to keep it up. He does, and before too long he nears his ideal weight. He buys new clothes, at least new pants with a smaller waist size. He does so well that he thinks he can stop eating the mail-order food and begin choosing on his own.

That is when the change begins to occur. As the weeks turn into months, he drifts back into his old eating habits. The weight returns, and now he is back where he started—seriously overweight. The saddest part is that he didn't improve his LDL cholesterol number while he was on his new diet. His prior victory is now only a fleeting memory. He lost weight but to no avail. There is a reason why his diet doesn't work and never will.

Mr. G. has been president of his company for about thirty years. He has been considered obese since high school. He always wears a suit and a tie. His face beams continuously. That is part of his success—his smile. He can win you over and close a deal and you feel happy about it because of that smile.

Mr. G.'s doctor informs him he is developing an elevated blood pressure and is prediabetic. Weight loss is recommended. There is a medical clinic in the city where he lives, and he is referred. There he is studied intensely with lab work, X-rays, and all the procedures that need to be performed for medical follow-up. A special diet is devised especially for him. Nutritionally, it is excellent. It has a certain percent of protein and a limit on fats and sugars. Over all, it results in fewer calories per day. He receives the food through the mail and eats it for the next year and a half.

He loses at least 80 percent of his excess weight. His face still beams. He continues being the business success he has been for years and is looking better and better. Then the day of success arrives. The medical clinic advises him he can stop ordering his food. He looks great. But two years later, he is almost back to his original weight. There is a reason why his diet doesn't work and never will.

The Secret to Losing Weight and Keeping It Off

I received a phone call from Jimmy Bob not too long ago. Jimmy Bob is a grammar school friend, and we have called each other from time to time ever since high school.

He called about some recent health problems his doctor had discussed with him. He mentioned he had gotten overweight and knew I had some ideas about what to do. He also had been told his LDL cholesterol was too high, and he had been placed on a statin. He wanted my advice. I went over the lifestyle strategies with him and gave him some encouragement.

He committed to losing his excess weight and getting his cholesterol-lowering drug to a smaller dose, hoping to get off it completely. He asked several questions concerning specifics of what he should not eat. He had been trying to lose some weight on his own, but the few pounds he had lost he had regained.

I was encouraged by what he was saying until he made a few revelations about how he was losing weight. A protein shake every morning for breakfast, multiple protein bars between meals, and six meals a day so he wouldn't overeat at any one meal.

"Am I on the right track?" he asked as innocently as a longtime friend could ask.

"I'm going to give you only one rule to follow."

"I'm listening."

"It is imperative that your sustaining weight diet is the same as your losing weight diet, or you will regain the weight."

Regaining lost weight is a failure.

I explained that if he was planning to lose weight and never regain it, he had to develop a proper eating lifestyle as he was losing his excess weight. "Only 2 to 20 percent of people who lose weight are able to sustain the loss," I explained. "Everybody else regains it, just like you did. The objective is to develop an eating plan that will allow you to maintain your weight once you reach your ideal weight. At that point, you will have developed a plan you can use for the rest of your life."

He was disappointed that he hadn't lost more weight on his homemade diet plan, which was a combination of what several of his friends were on. I told him not to worry about how much he lost but to concentrate on developing good eating habits.

The secret I shared with my friend is the most important thing I can say to you about weight loss: your sustaining weight diet has to be the same as your losing weight diet. If you develop proper eating habits as you lose weight, when you reach your ideal weight, you will have developed a lifestyle of eating that will allow you to maintain that weight. It is imperative that you lose weight by eating foods that will not increase your LDL cholesterol, and that you learn which foods will increase your HDL cholesterol.

Learning to eat properly is like practicing any other skill. The practice time comes during your weight-loss period. Practice, practice, practice. By the time you reach your ideal weight, you will be able to continue your healthy eating habits because you have restructured your thinking and your life.

Wouldn't it be great if you could sustain your ideal weight for the rest of your life? You can! No fad diet will do this. No supplement will give you success for years to come. No television ad can ensure that you will be able to sustain what you lose. You must use the time you are in the process of losing weight to practice and develop a permanent lifestyle of eating properly.

Eating healthy food to lose weight is of paramount importance because that is the same food you are going to eat as you maintain your weight the rest of your life.

Excess Weight and Your Heart

Medical literature reveals two key findings that help us understand the importance of getting to our ideal weight.

First of all, there is a direct correlation between being overweight and dying from heart disease. Second, there is a direct correlation between body weight and overall mortality.

In one study, researchers studied almost three thousand autopsies in Kentucky. They wanted to see if there was a correlation between being overweight and dying of heart disease. This was a fairly straightforward study dealing simply with weight. Researchers didn't determine if the deceased exercised or ate the wrong foods or what their LDL cholesterol was. Their question simply was, How many people who died from causes other than accidental death had blockages in the arteries of their heart, and what percent of those people were overweight? Of those who died from heart disease, 71 percent had an unhealthy BMI (Body Mass Index), which means they were overweight or obese.

Most people can understand how extra weight on a knee joint can lead to damage. But the joints in your body are not nearly as important as your heart. Look at the physiology of what happens to your heart because of excess weight. Whether you have ten pounds or a hundred pounds of extra fat on your body, your heart has to pump blood to that extra tissue to keep it alive. If you are overweight or obese, your heart has to work harder.

If you are supposed to weigh 150 pounds and you are "only" 15 pounds overweight, that is a 10 percent extra workload for your heart. As that extra weight increases, the volume of blood that your heart has to pump also increases.

If you could visualize what your body does to take care of extra fatty tissue, it would astonish you. First, miniature arteries begin to form. Then a new complex of arteries, veins, capillaries, and lymphatic drainage tubes begins to take shape to accommodate the extra blood flow. In turn, your heart generates higher pressures to pump an extra volume of blood to the extra tissue. This puts strain on your heart muscle. Depending on how overweight you are, there comes a time when the heart muscle just can't pump the extra amount of blood, and heart failure sets in.

There is a difference between placing an added workload on your heart by exercising and placing an extra workload on your heart by making it pump more blood volume than it normally does. When you exercise for thirty minutes and cause your heart to exert itself for that amount of time, the muscle fibers respond by increasing in size and strength. This is similar to your arm muscles increasing in size and strength when you lift weights. Your heart responds to that thirty-minute period of time and becomes stronger. However, if you place an extra workload on your heart twenty-four hours a day, your heart will become exhausted and will finally have to give up.

The initial physical sign of heart failure is swelling around the ankles. That lets you know your heart is failing to perform properly. Next, fluid accumulates in your lungs and you become short of breath. If something isn't done to correct the problem, your failing heart will quit beating.

A middle-aged man I once met comes to mind. He was a motivational speaker and often spoke to National Football League teams. He was as strong as an ox. His biceps were as big as my thigh muscles. He could impress the players with the amount of weight he could lift. He was probably the strongest person I had ever met. Over a few years, this impressive man grew—not in muscle mass but by putting on excess weight. He remained strong, but he added a lot of fat mass to his body, especially his abdomen.

I saw him about a year later. He was trim, and I wondered how he had gotten all the excess weight off.

"I was at my doctor. He told me I would have to lose weight or I was going to die. The doctor said it was one or the other. Lose weight or die. Period.

"He then told me there was a nursing home three blocks from his office, and he wanted me to go by and just look at the people there. The last statement he made to me was, 'You won't find any fat people there. They have all died.'"

My friend quit smiling. He got serious.

"I did just that. When I walked down the hall, I saw many people in wheelchairs, some sitting in the little game room playing cards or working on puzzles, and others in their rooms, lying in bed or sitting in a chair. My doctor was right. There were no fat people anywhere. They had all died. So I decided to get thin."

Visiting that rest home turned him around. He decided—and committed—to change his lifestyle of eating. He knew something about the foods he should eat but had a few questions. I explained that he shouldn't set a goal to lose weight in order to live long enough to get into a nursing home. His goal needed to be to lose weight in order to stay active and avoid the nursing home. "You want to be active when you die." I laughed, and so did he.

Being overweight is a disease. The good news is it is one you can cure yourself.

Your Health Retirement Plan

I know an individual who is a very joyful fellow. Everyone likes to be around him. He smiles a lot and is personable and fun. He is obese, but it doesn't seem to bother him in the least. When we are eating out together with friends, he makes a point of smiling at me as he spreads large amounts of butter onto his roll. "I really like butter," he says as he takes the first bite. His mind-set is, "I enjoy life. I enjoy eating. I am getting around like I want. I'm okay. I don't want to be able to run. I don't particularly want to jog. And I really don't want to live extra years in a nursing home." He takes a second bite and keeps smiling.

So what is wrong with enjoying life to its fullest right now? What is wrong with enjoying what you like to eat? And if you don't want to exercise, is that so bad? Especially if you don't enjoy exercising?

Most people think about retirement and the kind of life they want in the future. Businesses provide retirement plans so that when you get older you will have some money to enjoy life. The more you plan ahead and the more you save for the future rather than spend today, the better your retirement life will be. That makes sense from a financial standpoint to most people. You may have to give up a little of your enjoyment of the present, but the sacrifice will be worth it as you age. You may have to stay in a Holiday Inn rather than a Ritz Carlton on your vacation, but you will be able to go on a vacation after you retire rather than having to stay at home. You may have to buy a less expensive car and be satisfied with it, but you will have more money in the bank once you retire. Most people opt to have a retirement plan even if their financial planning means they have to give up something they want in the present for something greater they will enjoy in the future.

Have you ever thought about the single most important aspect of your retirement years? The odds are you have talked to your financial advisor about how much money you are going to have during that time. You have probably been contributing to your company's retirement fund. You may have even looked up what Medicare pays. Let me tell you what is much more important than the money aspect of retirement. It's something no 401(k) can provide. Your health. Your health is much more valuable than the amount of money in your retirement fund.

If you are planning only financially for your retirement, you are not really planning, because you may not be alive to enjoy retirement if you don't plan for better health. No matter how much money you will have, you won't be able to buy back your health. The younger you begin "health investing," the better. It is time to ask yourself about your health retirement plan. No matter how healthy you presently are, you can invest even more for tomorrow.

Making the decision and the commitment now to get your body into the best physical condition possible will be the best retirement investment you will ever make. And best of all, it won't cost you a penny.

▶ Action Steps

1. Place a notepad beside your television. Write down each time you see an advertisement concerning losing weight. Summarize the ad and put in writing why the weight lost will be regained 80 to 98 percent of the time with that program.

2. Eat a high-fiber cereal with three fruits daily for the next week. (Skipping the eggs and bacon will help your cholesterol numbers.)

3. Eat no desserts for the next two weeks.

4. Reaching Your Ideal Weight

As a physician, I'm troubled that people don't seem alarmed that over half of all Americans die from disease in their arteries. The medical reality is that being overweight plays a major role in these findings. Being overweight increases your lethal LDL cholesterol and lowers your hero HDL cholesterol. Being overweight is one of the worst things you can do to your body, yet two-thirds of us are either overweight or obese.

When I was in college, one of my premed professors stated, "Look at the student on your right side. The statistics show that either you or the student you just looked at will not make a good enough grade in this course to apply to medical school, much less get accepted."

I didn't want to believe him, but I realized that unless I studied as hard as I could and did everything possible to get an A, I might be the one who didn't get to apply to medical school. At that moment, I decided I wanted to be in the good 50 percent. I decided I was going to do all I could to make the grade.

The same thinking applies to your health. If you want to be in the 50 percent of people who do not die from disease in their arteries, you must decide to do everything possible to lose weight and lower your cholesterol. Getting to an ideal weight is one of the main factors in preventive medicine. Unless you take action to prevent the inevitable, you are headed for some rough years as you age and your health declines. If you get to your ideal weight, you not only will have a greater chance of living longer but also can begin having quality of life now. You can develop an active life that has meaning no matter how long that life may last.

You can lose excess weight. You are about to learn important steps that will help you get weight off and keep it off from now on. Don't wait for a heart attack to strike. You may not get a second chance to change your life. Grasp the opportunity to reach your ideal weight—whether you have only a few extra pounds or a hundred or more pounds to lose.

I got another call from Jimmy Bob not long ago. I can't remember talking to someone who was more excited. He was down to his goal weight. He and his wife had both changed their eating habits. His numbers were good. His doctor had taken him off most of the medication he had been on. He was feeling better than he had in years. He went on and on.

But the most exciting part of his call was when he told me he had shared his journey with three of our high school classmates, and they too had changed their lifestyles. During the next two months, I received emails from those classmates telling me how their lives were different. They were even getting their children and other friends on board. Now it is your turn.

BMI and Ideal Weight

The National Institutes of Health uses Body Mass Index (BMI), formulated using your height and your weight, as a measure of whether your weight is in a normal, overweight, or obese range. Normal is a BMI below 25, overweight is 25 to 30, and obese is over 30. The problem with these ranges is that they do not identify an ideal weight for a particular person. You can be thirty pounds above your ideal weight and still fall within the normal BMI range. This is because everyone is different. Some people are heavy boned or heavily built. Some are much more muscular than others, and muscle mass weighs more than fat tissue. Some are petite.

Being in the normal BMI range doesn't necessarily mean you are at your ideal weight. In fact, only 12 percent of Americans are at their ideal weight. But you can determine your ideal weight and set it as your goal weight. Getting to your ideal weight is the goal—not just being in the normal BMI range.

How to Figure Your Ideal Weight

I am often asked, "How do I figure my ideal weight?"

The formula I like best is not the BMI but one that fine-tunes it. I call it the Ideal Body Mass Index (IBMI). Here is how it works.

Men use 105 pounds as the base weight for five feet. For every inch they are over five feet, they add five pounds. Therefore, the ideal weight for a five-foot-seven-inch male would be 140 pounds.

Women use 95 pounds as the base weight for five feet. For every inch they are over five feet, they add four pounds.

Therefore, the ideal weight for a five-foot-seven-inch female would be 123 pounds.

Using the IBMI scale, you have to take into account personal body differences, and you may have to add pounds accordingly. For example, individuals who lift weights and have a large muscle mass may have to add ten to twenty pounds to their ideal weight because muscle weighs more than fat. The same applies for bone structure. Some people are larger boned than others. Figure your IBMI and then fine-tune it for your body build.

▶ **Action Steps**

1. After calculating your ideal weight, write your goal weight on a sticky note and place it in a prominent place where you can see it often, such as your wallet, purse, or bathroom mirror.

2. Abstain from eating any red meat for the next ten days.

3. If you don't have a daily exercise program, begin briskly walking thirty minutes a day six days a week.

5. Simple Steps for Losing Weight

Some herbal pills guarantee a 5 percent weight loss. Others will stimulate a portion of your brain to curb your appetite, making you not want to eat as much. But what really works from a medical standpoint?

I remember seeing a scale used to weigh medication to the exact milligram. The scale had two trays, one suspended on each side of the middle support. The pharmacist placed an exact metal weight on one tray and poured powdered medication onto the other tray until the needle moved to the middle of the scale. Both sides were equal.

Some of the things people do, thinking they are promoting good health, are similar to placing one ounce of "ideas that sound good" on one side of the scale and a hundred-pound bag of medical reality on the other. They equate the ounce of unproven theory with the hundred pounds of medical research. They would rather rely on a pill that works on a segment of their brain to make them feel full rather than accept the fact that fruits and vegetables fill them up with the least amount of calories. To develop a healthy weight lifestyle, you need to understand the real weights for the scale. So many times you actually believe you are doing great things to achieve a healthy life. Yet the pill you are taking or the special food you are eating, when weighed against medically sound studies of what works, is having minimal effect on improving your health. A pill alone is far from the answer.

In this chapter, you will learn how to lose excess weight. The reason this material is so important is because it applies whether you are obese or at your ideal weight. Even those at a normal weight fluctuate frequently. If you get on your scale one morning and realize you are a pound or two over your ideal weight, you can apply the principles in this chapter to get back to your goal weight. It is imperative you maintain your weight at the proper level.

The way to lose weight and maintain your ideal weight is not a diet plan. It is a lifestyle strategy. Following are simple steps for losing weight.

Count Food Rather than Calories

Physiologically speaking, the number of calories you take in versus the number you burn determines your weight. So how do you focus on losing excess weight without counting calories?

The answer is knowing which foods make you feel full on the fewest calories. Fiber, fruits, and vegetables contain the least amount of calories for a given portion size and make you feel full on the fewest calories. These should be staples in your meals every day.

Cut Out Snacks

It is imperative to cut out snacks—they are superfluous calories. Snacks are tempting and deceitful. A snack fulfills your desire for something sweet in midmorning while you justify that it is only 100 calories. You say to yourself, "That tasted so good I think I will eat one more." The same desire hits you that afternoon and again before you go to bed, and without thinking, you have eaten an extra 400 calories for the day.

When you are trying to lose weight, snacks may be the most difficult problem to overcome. Exercise the ten-minute factor to help eliminate snacks altogether. For ten minutes, don't eat the snack. Drink water or a zero-calorie beverage. Then do something to get your mind off the snack. Call a friend. Read your emails. Go for a walk. Get back to business. Do something. You will control both your stomach and your mind.

Be especially vigilant when you are tempted to sneak into the kitchen before bedtime for a few bites. Don't be fooled into thinking you deserve a snack because you went all day without indulging. Bedtime is the worst time to eat! The added calories will only turn into fatty tissue as you sleep. Keep the ten-minute factor in mind when the refrigerator calls at night.

To lose excess weight, completely abstain from snacks. Once you are at your ideal weight, if you want a snack, it will consist of fruits or nuts.

Don't Eat Dessert

"I *hardly ever* eat dessert." That is the usual response I get when I talk with someone about desserts. When I explain the difference between the losing weight part of the plan and the sustaining weight part, the person grasps the importance of abstaining from sweets. Once you reach your ideal weight, there may be some types of desserts you can eat. They will probably be different from the ones you eat now, but you will find a dessert that will not harm your arteries.

But during the weight-loss process, the rule of thumb is going to be no desserts. Period. Once you make that decision, once you commit to not eating dessert, it will become a steadfast rule you can adhere to. Once it is set in stone in your mind, the next time you are offered a dessert it will be easier for you to say, "No thank you. I'm good." Passing up dessert will get easier because you will place your choice on the scale and realize the benefit of not eating the dessert as well as the harm if you do. Once you convince your mind, once you are committed in your heart, you will be in charge of the battle.

Watch Portions

The instructor who taught me to fly years ago battled with weight. We talked about his struggle as we flew all over the country preparing for my instrument rating. Six months went by, and he called me one day and said, "Your plan worked. I thought I would let you know how much I appreciate what you taught me. The portion advice was a huge help. I would eat about a half portion, wait ten minutes, and realize I was full."

He continued by stating he had lost forty-five pounds and was down to what he weighed when he finished high school.

"I've held that weight for several months and am going to be there from now on."

I was so glad to hear he had taken my advice on portions. A good plan is to place a 60 to 70 percent portion on your plate for starters. You can always go back and get a little more, but if you wait ten minutes, you won't even desire the extra.

When eating at home, if you are hungry, it is easy to fill your plate with excess food. You think you will want to eat everything on your plate, and about three-fourths of the way through you don't even think about stopping. You eat whatever is on your plate. This is a habit, and you can change it. For starters, place less on your plate and remember that you can actually leave some food—no matter what your mother taught you.

This practice may be more difficult in a restaurant because the portions are too large. If you pay for all that food, you feel obligated to eat it. Try this simple tip. Stop two-thirds of the way through your meal and enjoy your tea or water or coffee and talk to the person you are eating with, or pull out your phone and check your emails if you are by yourself. Whatever you do, let some time pass, and your sense of fullness will come. Another trick is to stop eating halfway through your meal and ask for a take-home container for the remainder of your food. Just make sure what you choose for dinner will make a tasty and healthy lunch the next day.

There is a positive side to the portion plan. You can forget about portion sizes with fruits and vegetables. You can eat as many as you want, as long as they are not fried. Eating as many fruits and vegetables as you want at mealtime is permissible because there are fewer calories in these foods and you get a full feeling while eating them.

Don't Eat Fried Foods

Frying something adds about a third more calories to the food. Go grilled or baked.

Exercise

Your odds of losing weight and keeping it off are almost nil unless you develop a personal exercise program. The more exertion, the better, but even if your program begins with a simple brisk walk five days a week, it is a thousand times better than being sedentary. Exercise convinces your mind that you are serious about losing weight. It is a motivator that has no equal.

A Brown University study compared two groups of overweight women. One group dieted and exercised, while the other group only dieted. Those who dieted and exercised lost almost twice the amount of weight as those who did not exercise. I won't say you can't reduce your weight if you don't exercise, but such a statement isn't far from the truth. If you want to lose weight and keep it off, do more than just diet.

Be Accountable

I recently read that a person exercises more consistently if their spouse also exercises. How important is it to have an accountability partner or group? Would you eat better if you were in a group in which members kept everyone accountable for what they had for lunch? Would you be less likely to skip an exercise routine if you were supposed to meet someone at a particular time and place? What about a group challenge to lose a certain amount of weight by a set date?

Make yourself accountable to someone. It may be your spouse or a friend who has also realized the necessity of changing their lifestyle. Or it may be a group of people who want encouragement from others who are on the same pathway. Peer pressure works in mysterious ways. A recent study showed that individuals with an accountability partner lost 20 percent more weight than individuals who were also losing weight but did not have accountability partners.

Avoid Weight-Loss Supplements

I conclude this weight-loss portion with one of the saddest experiences I ever had in my medical practice. It deals with alternative treatments as compared to lifestyle changes.

Hardly a day goes by that I don't hear about, or get asked about, or read about, or see advertised some type of product that is supposed to make you look or feel younger. There are herbal medicines, Asian roots, special juices, and all types of mail-order drugs that help you lose weight or enhance your health in some way.

"Problems with the tips of fingers" was written on her chart. When I examined the female college student, my eyes were immediately drawn to the tips of all her fingers, thumbs included. They were as black as charcoal, and from the base of her fingernails to the tips of her fingers, the skin looked like wrinkled, dried black leather. It was evident she was not getting blood flow throughout the ends of her fingers.

I took her right hand into mine. As I held it, I felt for the pulse in her wrist. It was pounding. She had good blood flow into her hand, even in the small arteries along the side of each finger, but none in the tips.

I figured she must be on some type of medication that was overreacting with her system, causing those smallest of arteries located at the tips of her fingers to go into some type of spasm.

"Are you on any type of medication?" I asked.

"No." She looked at me and shook her head.

"You haven't been on any drugs?" She certainly didn't look like the kind who would take drugs. She was sweet. Had a pleasant smile. Dressed nicely. A little overweight.

"No, I have never taken drugs."

My mind raced through all the possibilities I could think of from a vascular surgeon's standpoint. I couldn't explain what was causing her problem.

"It's not a medicine, but I am taking a little capsule to lose weight. Five or six girls in my sorority are taking the same capsule. They don't have any trouble with their fingers. We are all losing weight. I have lost eight pounds myself."

The herbal compound was working for losing weight. But something else was also going on within her body. She had lost blood flow to the tips of all her fingers, and all ten were going to have to be amputated.

She had no idea of the cause. The capsules did not come with any type of warning. Her friends didn't have any trouble with their fingers. And they were all losing weight.

Unfortunately, many herbal supplements are not tested by the FDA. The first test is to make sure a medication causes no harm. If you want to lose weight, beware of alternative treatments. If there has not been a certified trial on a drug, beware.

Lose weight the medically sound way by taking charge of your weight-control lifestyle.

▶ Action Steps

1. Do not eat one bite of food between meals or after dinner for the next seven days (noncaloric liquid is okay).
2. Eat Fiber One cereal with three fruits and skim milk every morning for the next fourteen days.
3. Make a list of six vegetables you will begin eating at home and ordering when you eat out. Eat three of them today.
4. Go through your kitchen and throw out all cookies, processed meat, pastries, and candy. (If you were an alcoholic trying to quit, you wouldn't have any alcohol in your refrigerator or cabinets.)

PART 3

LIFESTYLE 2:
FOOD

6. Fats to Never Eat

You do not just want to add years to your life by eating properly. You want to add quality to those years. Who would want to live an extra seven to twelve years in a wheelchair or a bed or just sitting and staring at the wall? That is not what quality of life is about. The length of your life is important, but the quality is the ultimate factor. You want the last decade of your life to be quality years in which you are alert and active and no one is required to care for you. Those quality years can begin today and persist until your last day comes. Developing the proper eating lifestyle is one change you can make to ensure this important goal in your life.

If someone told you that you have over a 50 percent chance of dying from something preventable, would you take action to prevent it from happening? If you were standing in the middle of the road and an 18-wheeler was coming down the hill toward you, would you get out of the way? Or would you just stand there and let it run over you? Disease of your arteries is that truck.

I have traveled to villages in remote Africa and Papua New Guinea where the most primitive tribes left on earth live. I have operated on some of the people. My fingers have felt the arteries inside eighty-five-year-olds, and they were like the arteries of a ten-year-old. Soft and pliable. No plaque. No blockages. And these people do not have heart attacks or strokes. Why? What they eat keeps their blood cholesterol low. The diet in Africa consists mostly of dishes made from corn. Meat is eaten only on special occasions. In Papua New Guinea, about 95 percent of what they eat is some type of sweet potato. Studies of people in these tribes found that their average total cholesterol is 150. In America, people with a cholesterol of 150 simply don't have heart attacks. Foods from around the world teach us the benefits of low blood cholesterol. What follows will teach you how to get your blood cholesterol low—without having to plant a single sweet potato.

The quality of your life depends greatly on the foods you consume.

Genetics

Before we talk about food, we need to discuss genetics. Do genetics play a role in blood cholesterol? Do you blame your parents or the food you eat for your high cholesterol? A man I ate lunch with recently stated, "My genes are just bad for cholesterol. My wife eats the same as I do, and her cholesterol is lower than mine. I think it's just my genes." He said this as he took another bite of cheeseburger and wiped his lips with a napkin. He believed his high cholesterol wasn't his fault. I explained that he was partially correct, but only up to a point.

"Genes do make up 10 to 12 percent of the detriment, but the rest is up to you. What you inherit is not nearly as significant as your eating lifestyle." I spoke without interruption because he was busy eating. "The medical literature contains reports of people leaving one country, where they do not eat foods high in saturated fat, trans fat, and dietary cholesterol, and moving to America. Their blood cholesterol levels increase, resulting in a significant rise in the rate of heart attacks and strokes. One study showed that Japanese men who moved from Japan to California or Hawaii ended up with a much higher cholesterol level and a higher incidence of heart disease than Japanese men remaining in Japan. The ones who moved to the United States carried the same genes they had in Japan, but their eating lifestyles changed. They began eating steak and cheese and foods with butterfat in them. Ice cream became routine. And a large percentage of what they ate was fried.

"Their genes didn't make the difference. What they ate elevated their lethal LDL cholesterol levels," I explained while watching him eat his last two French fries.

"The important thing to remember is that if you do have bad genes, you need to be even more committed to controlling what you eat."

Bad Fats and Good Fats

The dangers of eating the wrong fats have been well publicized in recent decades. What does surprise people, though, is that there are actually good fats. If that excites you, keep reading.

Five or six women were standing around talking. I and two other husbands were off to the side in our own discussion. Even though I was listening to one of the men in our group,

I couldn't help but overhear what a woman from Switzerland was saying. She was explaining that she cooked dinner most every evening and was describing her cuisine to the other women. "I do a lot of French-style cooking," she was saying, "a lot of delicious sauces—cream sauces and pork loin and . . ." She went on for a while until one of the other women replied that it sounded good but contained a lot of fat.

"Oh, but fat is good for you," she exclaimed while leaning a little forward to make her statement. "It is essential for your bones. Fat also helps lubricate your joints. You need lots of fat. I know because my food doctor told me." She looked and sounded very authoritative.

In the United States, we tend to think all fats are bad. We don't usually acknowledge that certain fats are good and healthy. Yet in Switzerland, it must be the opposite. They must think all fats are good and obviously haven't learned about the bad ones. Especially if they want good bones and like to keep their joints working properly.

There are indeed bad fats you want to avoid like the plague, but there are also good fats. Good fats, those containing monounsaturated fat and polyunsaturated fat and omega-3 and omega-6 particles, not only decrease LDL cholesterol but also increase HDL cholesterol. Good fats are found in olives, nuts, avocados, and fish.

The *Journal of the American Heart Association* recently published one of the most significant reports concerning fats I have read. The article focused on the importance of getting healthy fats into one's diet. The study used diet information from 186 countries to see how eating certain fats affects the risk of heart attacks. Researchers found that about 10 percent of deaths from heart attacks were due to people eating too little of the healthy fats. This study showed not only the importance of not eating unhealthy fats but also the importance of eating healthy fats.

The Bad Fats to Avoid

When you are grocery shopping, allow a little extra time to examine the nutrition facts box on labels. Pay close attention to trans fat, dietary cholesterol, and saturated fat. These are the bad fats you want to avoid. Every time you check these items, you are reinforcing your knowledge of what foods can harm you now and in years to come.

Trans Fat

We have all heard about trans fat, but what is it really? First, it is the most dangerous fat we consume. The government has recently outlawed the use of trans fat and has given food manufacturers a three-year window to eliminate it from foods. However, in the future some of the same types of fat will still be used and labeled as hydrogenated or partially hydrogenated oil. It is used primarily as a preservative in prepackaged food that allows for a long shelf life. Trans fat, or hydrogenated oil, is absolutely the worst of the fats and must be avoided completely.

Dietary Cholesterol

Cholesterol is essential for the working of your body. Your liver is the source of the cholesterol that is in your bloodstream. The liver produces all the cholesterol your body needs every day. This is where LDL cholesterol and HDL cholesterol come from.

The cholesterol found in foods is different. It is called dietary cholesterol. It does not go directly into your bloodstream and does not turn into blood cholesterol. Egg yolk is the most common source of dietary cholesterol. Dietary cholesterol can cause the liver to produce extra cholesterol under certain conditions.

Every five years the US Department of Health reviews the dietary guidelines the government provides to help Americans live healthier lives. To do this, the Dietary Guidelines Advisory Committee reviews and evaluates current medical studies and reports on the findings. Sometimes the media interprets such reports a little differently than the committee intends. For example, here are the kinds of newspaper headlines you might have seen when a recent report came out.

"New Dietary Guidelines Reverse Recommendations on Cholesterol"

"Nutrition Panel Calls for Less Sugar and Eases Cholesterol and Fat Restrictions"

"Ending the War on Fat"

Such statements from the media make it seem as if you don't have to be concerned about your blood cholesterol or avoiding bad fats anymore. But that is not what the committee said.

If you read the summary of the Dietary Guidelines Advisory Committee, you will find that their advice is similar to what is being recommended here. The committee stated that the overall body of evidence suggests that the healthiest dietary pattern is higher in vegetables, fruits, whole grains, low- or nonfat dairy, seafood, legumes, and nuts and lower in red and processed meat. The list identified as detrimental included sugar-sweetened foods and beverages as well as refined grains. One of the most important takeaways from the studies reviewed by the committee is that people should limit their intake of saturated fat. The committee agreed.

The committee made one change that is at odds with the plan described in this book. The committee took dietary cholesterol off the list of foods to avoid. As already noted, the main source of this type of cholesterol is egg yolk. It is true that dietary cholesterol is not as bad on your arteries as saturated fat. However, even if dietary cholesterol is removed from the discussion, egg yolk still contains more saturated fat than is acceptable on our program.

The American Heart Association's dietary recommendations say, "Limit foods high in saturated fat, trans-fat, and cholesterol." A Mayo Clinic cardiologist responded in a newsletter to the question, "Are chicken eggs good or bad for my cholesterol?" He answered that if you are healthy, you should consume no more than 300 mg of cholesterol a day. If you have diabetes, high cholesterol, or heart disease, you should limit your daily cholesterol intake to no more than 200 mg a day. He went on to point out that if you like eggs but don't want the extra cholesterol, you should use only the egg whites or use cholesterol-free egg substitutes, which are made with egg whites.

Other medical reports state that if you are diabetic, the consumption of egg yolks increases your chances of developing cardiovascular disease. None of the medical reports list egg yolks as a health food.

In this book, we are focused on prevention. If avoiding a certain food will help you avoid diabetes, elevated blood cholesterol, or heart disease, why would you wait until you have one of these conditions to take action? For me to recommend that you avoid dietary cholesterol only after you have developed diabetes or high blood cholesterol or heart disease would be similar to me advising one of my lung cancer patients to quit smoking after the diagnosis. It would be good to do but a little late.

Rather than relying on media headlines, look at the medical literature when making decisions on how you are going to develop your eating lifestyle. I encourage you to evaluate your food choices from the prevention angle. Don't tempt yourself to eat something that has saturated fat, like egg yolks, especially if that food is associated with bacon and gravy and buttered toast and other foods that you also want to avoid.

Saturated Fat

Saturated fat is the number one food item to avoid. This bad fat is found in more kinds of food than any of the other bad fats. If I were to pick one substance for you to check on every food item you buy, it would be saturated fat.

The Food and Drug Administration or the American Heart Association or most any other organization that studies how certain foods harm the body recommends that you limit saturated fat to a certain percentage of your intake each day. Such organizations may state you should limit saturated fat to 10 percent of your total food intake daily.

Does anyone keep track of the amount of saturated fat they eat throughout a day? I have never met anyone who keeps such a record. Common sense tells me to avoid food with saturated fat 100 percent of the time.

Learn which foods contain saturated fat so you can avoid them. Foods with saturated fat are the cause of the formation of LDL splinters, which result in inflammation and blockage of your arteries. The goal is to eat zero saturated fat.

If you pick up a bag of potato chips and read in the nutrition facts box that it contains 1.5 g of saturated fat per serving, put it back. Look a few bags down the aisle and find the baked potato chips that have 0 g of saturated fat. Put that bag in your cart. You want to eat foods that contain between 0 g and 0.5 g of saturated fat.

Years ago, I read an article in the medical literature concerning saturated fat that changed my eating habits for life. It stated that the saturated fat in the foods we eat is the main cause of the formation of the bad LDL cholesterol in our blood. The article also pointed out that over half of Americans die of a heart attack or a stroke because of blockages in their arteries resulting from excess LDL cholesterol floating around in their bloodstreams.

I had to acknowledge the medical facts concerning LDL cholesterol's negative effect on my arteries. Then I read the rest of the article. It stressed that we get most of our saturated fat from cheese. Cheese doesn't necessarily have the highest content of saturated fat, but we eat so much of it that it ends up being the source of the largest amount of saturated fat we consume.

At that time, cheese was my favorite food. My friends knew that. My patients knew that. They would give me all kinds of cheese for Christmas. I would eat them for months. However, as I finished reading that article, I decided then and there to quit eating cheese. To me, it was black and white. Why would I keep eating any food, even my favorite, if it were going to cause my arteries to become inflamed and blocked? I made part of my living cleaning plaque out of blocked arteries. I already knew the consequences. That very week I had operated on a man who had experienced a stroke six weeks prior because of blockage in one of the arteries that carries blood to the brain. I had held the piece of plaque in my gloved hand. I had hollowed it out of the wall of his artery like a pea out of its pod. Why would I knowingly eat food that caused such a problem?

It was difficult to abstain from cheese at first, but it became easier and easier as I reminded myself that saturated fat causes an increase in LDL cholesterol and what that does to my arteries. The following Christmas my patients still brought me cheese. I filled the table in the office kitchen and told all the employees about the article I had read. I explained that they shouldn't eat it, but it was their choice. They could have my Christmas cheese.

Make the decision to begin improving your health by avoiding bad fats, resolving that you want to live younger longer.

The Evils of Rationalization

A woman asked me a very good question the other day. "I read that hard cheese is not as bad for you as other cheeses. It would be helpful to limit your eating to just those special cheeses, wouldn't it? I think they come from Switzerland."

Her husband, who happened to be a physician, jumped right into the conversation. "I am sure you are aware that the small LDL cholesterol particles are the ones that do the most damage to our arteries." He didn't allow me to respond before moving on to the point he wanted to make. "I read that cooking steak on the grill is more dangerous because there are more small LDL particles. That's why I eat my steak rare." He smiled. "Not raw, but very rare. And I try to eat only grass-fed beef."

They had both fallen into a trap so many people fall into when they attempt to appease themselves. I call it the evils-of-rationalization trap.

My response was to point out the fallacy of their thinking. "You have to realize that cheese and red meat contain lots of saturated fat. Also know that food is an addiction." I looked initially at the wife. "If you try to eat only a special type of cheese, such as a hard cheese from Switzerland, your desire for cheese in general will remain the same. It may even increase. In trying to teach your mind not to want the foods that contain saturated fat that will harm your arteries, you have to wipe out your desire for those foods. If you eat the special cheese, you will eventually go back to eating any cheese.

"As far as eating red meat not cooked as warm, the same answer applies." I wasn't going to argue with either of them about whether hard cheese is not as bad as other cheese or whether overcooking your steak is worse than eating rare meat. But I did want to get them thinking about a good plan to follow if they really had a desire to improve their lifestyle of eating. I ended with my favorite gnat illustration. "Just remember that when you begin focusing on small details, most of the time you think you are shooting at elephants but you are actually only killing gnats." They both laughed and agreed they probably needed to face the reality about saturated fat.

Much is also coming out in the media concerning sugar. Books are being written stating that it is not fat that causes heart attacks and plaque in your arteries but sugar. The problem with such reports is that they contain 80 percent truth and then take off on a tangent to get a point across concerning how bad sugar is for your body. I read a book of Mark Twain's quotations, and one I like relates to what I am saying about such reports. He said that a particular someone he knew always told the truth . . . but not always the strict truth. I am afraid some media articles we read don't tell us the strict truth.

The media may report that fat is not bad for you; sugar is the problem. "Go ahead and enjoy the fat," they say. "Just stay away from the sugar."

First, remember the medical truth about fats. Bad fats cause damage to arteries, causing more heart attacks and strokes. Saturated fat is the kind you eat the most that causes you harm.

Do not fall into the trap of lumping bad fats into the category of fats in general. The medical literature does not do this, and you shouldn't either. Bad fats are the reason doctors prescribe statin medications to lower LDL cholesterol. As you already know, bad fats cause LDL cholesterol to be elevated. Numerous studies have made this connection, and numerous studies have shown that if you lower your LDL cholesterol with lifestyle changes, you will have less chance of having a heart attack or a stroke.

Further studies have shown that if people stop eating bad fats but substitute extra sugar in their place, the heart attack numbers do not improve. When bad fats are avoided and replaced with good fats, fruits and vegetables, nuts, peas, beans, and fish, there is a significant decline in heart attacks and strokes.

The take-home message is this: avoid red and processed meats, cheese, butter, cream, fried foods, and foods that contain much saturated fat. When you stop eating the foods containing the bad fats, don't replace them with extra-sugar foods. Don't go to the donuts, cookies, candy, and sweet desserts. Instead, replace bad fats with good ones, plus fruits, vegetables, salmon, tuna, avocados, and nuts, and use olive oil and canola oil instead of animal-based frying oils.

Don't rationalize your choices and think you can reward yourself with a big piece of chocolate cake just because you didn't eat a steak.

▶ Action Steps

1. Go to your cupboard and spend ten minutes looking for saturated fat on the nutrition facts boxes.

2. Evaluate the nutrition facts box on every item you intend to purchase in the grocery or convenience store this week. Keep track of how many items you put back because of what you have learned.

3. Choose baked chips instead of regular chips.

4. Buy a bottle of good fat olive oil or canola oil today. Throw out any animal-based oil you have in your kitchen.

7. Foods to Avoid at Each Meal

Now that you know about the bad fats, we can discuss the foods you should avoid at each meal.

The Bad Breakfast

Bacon, Sausage, and Eggs

Open a breakfast menu at any restaurant and you will see the most common food offerings include eggs with bacon or sausage. Remember that egg yolk has more saturated fat than is optimal in our plan. One yolk exceeds the daily saturated fat limit. Plus, there is a correlation between processed meats such as bacon and sausage and an increase in LDL.

Biscuits

Biscuits will also need to go. Many of the biscuits at restaurants are made using lard or similar food substances that cause LDL cholesterol to increase.

I got to watch biscuits being made at a popular fast-food restaurant. Biscuits are their bestseller. The first step involved opening a package of lard three inches wide, three inches high, and twelve inches long. On the top of the lard package were small blue marks about an inch apart. The biscuit maker took a knife and sliced the lard at each blue line. Each hunk was used to make a certain number of biscuits. As I watched, I couldn't help but think to myself how similar the lard was to the soft plaque I had taken out of the carotid arteries of patients. (You can see how much easier it is for a vascular surgeon to avoid certain foods.)

Whole Milk and Coffee Creamers

What about coffee? It doesn't contain anything that causes an increase in LDL, but most coffee creamers do. Avoid them.

What about the milk you drink at breakfast or pour on a bowl of cereal? Are dairy products bad for you? In the old days, you would buy a quart of milk and the top portion would be the cream. Today the pasteurizing process mixes that cream throughout the entire carton of milk. You can't see it, but it is there in whole milk. Whole milk contains about 4 percent butterfat. That translates into 6 g of saturated fat on the nutrition facts label. (Remember, you want to eat foods that contain between 0 g and 0.5 g of saturated fat.)

Skim milk has all the fat removed. It doesn't take a genius to figure this one out: if you want to decrease the amount of saturated fat you put into your body, begin using skim milk (or almond milk or soy milk) on a routine basis.

I recall when I first realized how much bad fat is in whole milk. I had never thought about it until I read that the fat in a glass of whole milk is equivalent to that in five strips of bacon. I couldn't even imagine how much fat is in a half gallon of whole milk.

I told my wife about all the saturated fat in milk and asked her to buy skim milk the next time she went to the grocery store. I will never forget the first morning I poured it on my cereal. It tasted like water. I got it down but did not like it at all. But I kept thinking about those five fatty bacon slices, and it wasn't long before skim milk began tasting normal. And soon a sip of whole milk made me wonder why I ever liked it in the first place.

When you think of whole milk, remember all the cream. You don't see it in today's milk, but it is there.

Butter

Last but not least, we have to address butter. Restaurants automatically put it on your toast at breakfast, on your baked potato at lunch, and into your sauces at dinner.

Is a pat of butter on your toast at breakfast all that bad? Remember, we are talking about an eating lifestyle. Eating habits. Eating addictions. If you make a habit of placing butter on your bread, you don't even think about it. If you have always placed a glob of butter on your baked potato, you will do it again the next time you eat one.

Make a habit of not eating the bad. Butter falls into the bad fat category. Margarine has about an equal amount of saturated fat as butter. Quit using both. Instead, use substitutes like Benecol or Promise Active. These are cholesterol-lowering spreads. Or eat your toast dry or put some of your favorite jam on it.

The Bad Lunch

Cheese

Ham and cheese sandwich. Double cheeseburger. French fries with melted cheese on top. Pita chips with cheese dip. Cheese sticks. Cheese pizza. Even if you order a salad, it most likely comes with cheese on it unless you ask for it to be left off.

People tell me it is harder for them to give up cheese than any other bad fat foods. I assure you it will be easier to develop the eating lifestyle you need and want if you learn what cheese is doing to your health. You don't have to become a vascular surgeon and dig plaque out of an artery to make your decision. The more you know medically, the brighter those warning lights will become. Your eating habits will change.

I recently had lunch with a pediatrician who is thirty-nine years old. After I ordered grilled fish and he ordered meat with cheese sauce, he pointed out that this restaurant had very good cheese sauces. When he ordered his dessert, a chocolate cream cake with ice cream, he asked why I got only a cup of decaf coffee and no dessert. He pointed out that the dessert he ordered was one of the specialties of that restaurant.

I took a few minutes to explain how certain foods such as cheese cause inflammation and plaque in arteries. Before I could finish my little dissertation, he interrupted me with his view of what I was saying.

"I'm in love with cheese, and I'll tell you right now why I am going to enjoy eating everything I want. I don't want to live to be ninety. I think seventy-two or seventy-three will be just fine with me." He stared right at me. "My grandmother lived to be ninety, and the last eight years of her life were horrible. She couldn't get around and was sick a lot of the time. She ended up with dementia. She didn't know anyone. I will be happy to enjoy life now, die earlier, and not have to go through all the trouble she went through when she aged."

He made his point. Actually, it was an excellent lead into what I wanted to explain to him. Eating healthy is not about length of life but quality of life. I wanted to explain how he could develop lifestyles now that would give him active, quality years as he aged. I wanted to tell him but then realized he was the type that just wouldn't understand.

The only response that came to mind was one my older brother used to say to me when he knew he was right and I was wrong. So without further thought, I responded, "You may be right—but I doubt it."

Fried Foods

Fried chicken. Fried fish. French fries. Fried okra. Fried green tomatoes. The second group of bad foods for lunch includes anything fried.

Is it possible to eat no fried foods? That won't be a 100 percent rule, depending on what the food is fried in, but you should come as close to it as possible. Once you acknowledge what is causing your aging process, it will become easier for you to avoid fried foods.

The reason fried foods are bad is because most of them are fried in animal fat rather than in olive oil or canola oil. Animal fat is high in saturated fat. Plus, whenever you fry a food, you add about a third more calories.

Whether you are cooking at home or ordering at a restaurant, develop a habit of choosing grilled rather than fried foods. If you order grilled food rather than fried, you still have to be aware of the type of sauces they place on top of your grilled fish or chicken. So many of the sauces are cream or cheese based and contain as much fat as you would have eaten if the food had been fried. A good rule of thumb is simply to tell your server to place the sauces on the side. Then don't eat them. If you are cooking at home, use oils that are high in the good fats. The good fats are monounsaturated fat, polyunsaturated fat, and omega-3 fatty acids. They are found in canola oil and olive oil.

A third less calories and less LDL cholesterol are two good reasons not to eat fried foods. A baked potato is healthier than fries and grilled chicken is better than fried. Plus, I really do believe tomatoes taste better if they are not fried.

Cream-Based Soups

Cream of tomato soup. Oyster bisque. Clam chowder. Cream-based soups are a bad choice. The next time you order soup ask if it is cream based. It will surprise you how many are. The good news is there are plenty to choose from that don't have the cream.

If you are making soup at home, add skim milk or almond milk rather than whole. Or better yet, make a soup that is broth based.

The Bad Dinner

Salad Condiments

Many salads automatically come with saturated-fat-filled cheese on top. Whenever you order a salad, simply instruct your server to leave off the cheese. The same goes for the bacon bits and the crunchy fried noodles.

Salad Dressings

Always ask for the dressing to be placed on the side. Also ask for fat-free dressing. If eating a good salad is in your eating plan, don't negate the benefit by eating a dressing loaded with fat.

Red Meat

During an interview recently, I was asked if people should never eat red meat again. I explained the concept of food addiction. Eating a steak now and then is not going to cause you to die ten years earlier. The problem is that the desire for that steak can persist.

Frequently, I hear statements such as, "I eat red meat only in moderation" or "I eat red meat only once a week." My response is the usual no-brainer question. "If you were trying to eliminate your desire for cigarettes, would you let yourself smoke just on Saturdays? In moderation?" That usually gets a smile and a nod. "Only on Saturday" moderation will keep your desire for that weekend reward in your mind through-out the week. Sooner or later, your desire will cause you to give in to the temptation of red meat more often. Before you know it, you are frequently eating a food high in saturated fat that causes your LDL cholesterol to become elevated. Eating in moderation does not help you create and sustain your desired eating lifestyle.

A good rule of thumb is to decide not to eat any red meat. If you are invited to dinner somewhere and that is the only meat offered, go ahead and eat some. You are not trying to be fanatical. You are trying to avoid eating hamburgers and hot dogs and steak four or five times a week and trying to substitute grilled fish or chicken for your addiction.

If someone were addicted to alcohol and wanted to quit, you wouldn't suggest they drink only occasionally. If you did, the day would come when they were drinking routinely without any commitment to stop drinking. Just remember that food is an addiction, and the only way to break that addiction is through abstinence.

Don't be like the woman who had no desire whatsoever to give up red meat.

"I like steak. I don't think I could give it up." That is what she told me.

I quickly explained the medical facts that saturated fat causes an elevation of the lethal LDL cholesterol in her blood and that these particles are like little splinters that get into the walls of her arteries, causing inflammation and plaque formation resulting in heart attacks and strokes.

I went on to say that eating red meat not only increases her overall risk of disease in the arteries of her heart but also causes an increased risk of certain cancers. I even went over a study from the *Archives of Internal Medicine* of over a half million people that showed that men who ate the equivalent of a quarter-pound hamburger a day had a 22 percent higher risk of dying from cancer and a 27 percent higher risk of dying from heart disease than the men whose diets did not contain red meat. She appeared to be accepting the information, so I continued.

I explained that the study also showed what happened when the people who ate red meat changed their eating lifestyles and stopped eating such foods. There was an 11 percent decrease in mortality in the men and a 21 percent decrease in the women who changed to a healthy diet.

Lastly, I pointed out that this same study showed that total cholesterol and LDL cholesterol levels decreased in people who substituted fish for red meat.

I told this woman, "I grew up eating red meat. I never thought I would give it up. But the more I read and realized what it was doing to me, the easier it became to give up such food. I liked steak also, just like you do now. I didn't think I could give it up either. But I did."

I hope I convinced her, and I hope I convinced you.

Sauces

A "side" note. When you order a meal, ask the waiter to place the sauce on the side. Most sauces contain a lot of saturated fat, but you can make the decision whether to eat it after you see what it is. If you are not sure whether it is acceptable, a good rule of thumb is to avoid it.

Desserts

Do you have to give up desserts altogether? The answer during your weight-loss phase is yes. The answer during your weight-sustaining plan is mostly yes. While your friends are eating dessert, sip a cup of coffee and enjoy their friendship. However, you can find some healthy desserts you will come to enjoy eating occasionally, such as fat-free yogurt and angel food cake with strawberries, plus a multitude of fruits and nuts. My wife makes a tasty apple crunch dessert. It's a mixture of sliced apples, pecans, walnuts, and almonds.

She adds some maple syrup, cinnamon, nutmeg, and ginger and bakes it.

I have already told you about my addiction to cheese. My other addiction was ice cream. There is 4 percent butterfat in the cream in whole milk. That 4 percent multiplies when you concentrate that cream into ice cream. The butterfat in the choicest ice creams gets very high. (Before I quit eating ice cream, my favorite was 18 percent butterfat.)

It is difficult for physicians to encourage their patients to do something they are not doing themselves. I could not tell patients they should give up ice cream. It is difficult for an overweight doctor to explain to patients that they need to lose weight. I framed a cartoon once and placed it in my office. It depicted a markedly obese doctor sitting behind his desk, with an overweight patient sitting in a chair facing him on the other side of the desk. The doctor is pointing his finger toward the patient and saying, "You have got to go on a diet."

I could relate to that cartoon because I needed to go on a diet myself, one that eliminated ice cream altogether. I liked ice cream a lot. I ate it several times a week. I would fix a bowl and eat it while sitting on the sofa watching Monday Night Football. It was a part of me. My favorite flavor was crunchy caramel. But then I had one of those moments when I realized I needed to quit eating it.

I saw fat-free yogurt advertised and decided to replace ice cream with yogurt. That worked for several months until I was offered homemade ice cream at someone's house. They had a choice of chocolate or caramel syrup to top it off.

I couldn't resist. I ate only a small bowl, but the desire for a large helping was just as great as it had been months and years before. That evening I realized that certain foods are more than a habit. They are an addiction.

Once I realized this, I knew I had to beat the desire for the foods I adored. I had to quit eating the yogurt as well as the ice cream in order to break the desire and beat my addiction. After a couple of months, the desire began to leave. Eventually, I even could watch Monday Night Football without my usual treat.

Do you think you can go eight weeks without eating any dessert? Try it.

A Summary of Foods to Avoid

Breakfast
> Bacon and sausage
> Egg yolks
> Biscuits
> Whole milk and coffee creamers
> Butter

Lunch
> Cheese
> Fried foods
> Cream-based soups

Dinner
> Salad condiments
> Salad dressings
> Red meat
> Sauces
> Desserts

Remembering What Foods to Avoid

I had just finished eating lunch and was leaving the restaurant when a man I knew came up to me and said he was interested in learning what foods he should avoid to protect his health. I told him he wanted to avoid foods that contain saturated fat, trans fat, and dietary cholesterol. In less than two minutes, I painted him a mental picture of foods to avoid. The picture consisted of six categories, beginning with a juicy steak on a plate. Next came a fried egg on top of the steak and then a thick slice of cheese. To the right of the plate was a glass of whole milk, and to the left was a small pat of butter. Last was grease poured over the entire plate of food.

"This picture will help you remember about 90 percent of the foods you are going to eliminate from your eating lifestyle." He thanked me, and I proceeded out the door, wondering if my short explanation would help him.

I saw him in a group of people two days later, and he quickly walked over to me. "Last night I got to thinking about what you explained concerning the danger of saturated fat, trans fat, and dietary cholesterol. I just want you to know what I did. I took a gallon container of ice cream out of my freezer and threw it in the trash." After telling me the brand, he said, "It was my favorite ice cream. I ate it almost every night. But I threw it away." He laughed and walked back to the group he was with. "Just wanted you to know." He looked back at me and nodded one more time. He didn't even give me a chance to reply.

It is so exciting to see individuals make a commitment to change a part of their lives, especially when it involves throwing away a favorite ice cream they have eaten almost nightly for years. One thought ran through my mind as I walked away. His favorite ice cream was 28 percent butterfat. That realization made me feel even better.

▶ Action Steps

1. Eat a baked potato rather than French fries for a month. No butter or sour cream. (I fix mine by smashing it with a fork and pouring on a little olive oil as well as sprinkling pepper on top.)
2. Drink skim milk instead of whole milk.
3. Abstain completely from cheese, cream cheese, and cheese sauce on any food for the next two weeks.
4. Abstain from eating red meat for the next seven days.

8. The Good Food Platform

You have learned some of the main foods to avoid. Now let's look at the foods that are good for you, that build your health. The food recommendations below focus on both good foods and good fats. Build basic menus for each meal using both.

The Good Breakfast

Foods High in Fiber

Fiber is one of the best things you can eat for a good intestinal tract. Not only does fiber help protect you from colon cancer, but it also improves bowel movements. A high-fiber breakfast keeps you regular. Fiber regulates your bowels because fiber is not easily absorbed. It moves through your intestines quickly and at the same time absorbs water in your colon, making your stools softer and causing less straining. If you do not eat enough fiber, your stools become hard and you can become constipated.

Without the straining associated with constipation, there is less buildup of pressure within your colon that commonly results in small pouches in the wall of the colon. These little out-pouches are about as large as the end of your little finger and are called diverticula. These can easily become infected, resulting in what is called diverticulitis. These out-pouches can even rupture after becoming infected and require surgery. The *British Medical Journal* reported that those who eat more than 25 g of fiber a day have a 41 percent reduced risk of being hospitalized or dying of diverticulitis complications when compared to individuals who eat less than 14 g of fiber daily. The medical literature emphasizes that eating fiber is the best protection against diverticulosis and diverticulitis.

If you look at the nutrition facts on boxes of cereal, it is easy to pick out which ones contain the highest fiber content. The one that is consistently highest in fiber content is Fiber One. Most common cereals have 2 to 4 g of fiber, whereas Fiber One has 14 to 16, depending on which type you choose. A good alternative for a high-fiber breakfast includes steel-cut oats. Steel-cut oats have the outer covering intact for extra fiber. Whole-grain toast, without butter, is also a source of fiber.

Foods that have a high fiber content, like whole grains, cereals, and fruits are free of saturated fats. Therefore, eating high fiber cereal with added fruit for breakfast instead of bacon and eggs with biscuits and gravy is a great way to begin your day by lowering your LDL cholesterol.

Skim Milk

Instead of whole milk, use skim milk with zero saturated fat. Almond milk, soy milk, and rice milk also contain no saturated fat, so your LDL cholesterol will not become elevated.

Fruits

Any medical journal article about what foods you should eat will mention fruit. This is one food you should include or increase in your daily eating habits. Most people will occasionally eat fruit, but the emphasis now is to eat fruit daily. Breakfast is an easy way to start the day with fruit. Adding strawberries, bananas, blueberries, or raspberries to your cereal is an easy and tasty habit to acquire.

Egg Whites

Next on the breakfast menu is an egg white and veggie omelet. There are two reasons not to eat the egg yolk. One is the amount of saturated fat in it, and the other is the amount of dietary cholesterol in it. Egg yolk has the most concentrated amount of dietary cholesterol of any food we commonly eat. The American Heart Association recommends that if you have diabetes, high cholesterol, or heart disease, you should limit your daily cholesterol intake to no more than 200 mg. Since you are developing an eating lifestyle of prevention, be proactive and limit your dietary cholesterol before you develop diabetes, high blood cholesterol, or heart disease.

The Good Lunch

Fruits and Vegetables

Time and again, the medical literature highlights two food groups as healthy choices: fruits and vegetables.

Why do fruits and vegetables always make the list? Why are they always discussed in connection with losing weight? First, fruits and vegetables make you feel full with the fewest calories. But even more important is the fact that fruits and vegetables are nearly void of the bad fats that cause an elevation in LDL cholesterol.

It is easy to incorporate fruits and vegetables into your diet by eating a salad for lunch. A salad that includes peas, beans, and nuts is a good choice.

Chicken and Fish

For a sandwich, use grilled fish or chicken. If you order a sandwich at a fast-food restaurant, ask for no mayonnaise or cheese. Or add grilled fish or chicken to your salad.

Anytime you can get some type of fish for lunch, as long as it is not fried, order it. Fish contains the good omega-3 fat that helps increase your HDL cholesterol and lower your LDL. Eating fish three to five times a week is a good goal.

I want to point out that it is fish, not fish oil supplements, that has been shown to be a significant factor in reducing the risk of heart attacks. So don't depend on supplements. Eat the whole fish.

The Good Dinner

Salad

For most people, dinner is the main meal of the day. It usually begins with a salad, followed by the main course and then possibly a dessert. Your new lifestyle will certainly differ from that of most others, but beginning with a salad is still a good start. Whether at home or in restaurants, there are many salad combinations to choose from. Again, choose a nonfat dressing to avoid hidden saturated fat.

Fish

Grilled fish is still the emphasis. Eating fish three or more times a week is a good goal. I can't stress enough how important it is to eat the healthy fat found in fish. Fish is the double-barreled shotgun in fighting disease of the arteries. It lowers the unhealthy LDL and raises the healthy HDL.

When you order grilled fish in a restaurant, remember to ask your server to place the sauce on the side so you can determine whether it is cream or cheese based, which you will want to leave off. Salmon is probably the best choice and is found in most restaurants and grocery stores. Other fish such as tuna and trout also contains the good fat, as do lobster and shrimp.

Whole-Grain Pasta or Cheese-less Pizza

For something different, whole-grain pasta is a good alternative. There are habits you need to develop when ordering anything Italian. Rather than cheese or meat sauces, ask for simple tomato-based marinara. With whole-grain pasta, you are not only avoiding saturated fat but also eating the high fiber you need for your intestines.

Let me mention one treat my wife and I enjoy occasionally. We order it at a small restaurant that specializes in pizza, and they know what we want when we walk in. Our server just smiles and nods her head. The pizza she brings has no cheese, just the usual marinara that comes on all the pizzas. But on top of the thin, crispy crust are some pieces of Cajun spicy chicken, strips of fresh pineapple, and caramelized onions. If you try, you can get very creative with a cheese-less pizza.

These suggestions are a good start for your journey. You will discover additional foods you can use to fine-tune your meals, but right now begin making changes that will make a difference in how you spend the rest of your life.

Snacks

Let's talk about snacks for a minute. During the weight-loss phase of your new eating lifestyle, you should eat no snacks at all. Remember that even good snacks contain calories. These are essentially extra calories that will add on weight.

Snacks are permissible once you reach your ideal weight. The best snack choices are fruits or nuts. Again, fruits fill you up with few calories. Nuts are a good choice because they contain the good monounsaturated fat that raises your HDL cholesterol. They do contain some saturated fat, but the large amount of good fat outweighs the bad. Walnuts and almonds are some of the best, but if you eat any kind of nut for a snack rather than an Oreo cookie, you have made a better choice.

A Summary of Foods to Eat

Breakfast
    Foods high in fiber
    Skim milk
    Fruits
    Egg Whites

Lunch

    Fruits and vegetables

    Chicken and fish

Dinner

    Salad

    Fish

    Whole-grain pasta or cheese-less pizza

Snacks

    Fruits

    Nuts

Your Food Lifestyle

Don't kid yourself when dealing with your most prized possession: your health. There are many ways we rationalize when it comes to eating. "I will eat only half a slice of that butter-filled cake," you tell yourself. "Moderation is the rule I am going to live by," you say. "I bought this at the organic food store, so it must be all right for me to eat." The list goes on and on.

As you begin your new lifestyle journey, keep your eating habits simple. Learn to differentiate between basic good foods and bad ones. Learn to choose good fats over bad ones. Recognize the difference between the bad saturated fat and the good monounsaturated and polyunsaturated fats. This knowledge will help you choose cereal over bacon, eggs, and biscuits for breakfast; a grilled chicken sandwich over a cheeseburger and fries for lunch; and fish over steak for dinner. Base your eating habits on the medical reality of what foods do to your cholesterol, your weight, and the aging process of your body.

▶ Action Steps

1. Eat the good fat in grilled fish at least twice this week.
2. Eat a salad for lunch. Add grilled chicken or fish if you like. Choose a fat-free salad dressing.
3. Eat nothing fried for a week.

9. Cancer-Causing Foods

Food has a significant impact on the health of arteries, but it also plays a role in increasing the likelihood of certain cancers. It is important to know what the medical literature says about ways you can help prevent certain cancers in relation to the foods you eat.

When learning which foods to avoid and which to eat in order to keep control of your cholesterol, it becomes a real serendipity to realize the foods that are bad for your cholesterol are also the ones to avoid to help prevent certain cancers. Colon cancer is one of those cases. Eating red meat causes your LDL cholesterol to increase. That same food also has an effect on cancer of the colon.

Recently, the World Health Organization reported the significant harmful correlation between processed meats and red meat and colon cancer. Processed meat is meat that has been changed in some way to affect taste or increase shelf life. Processed meats include bacon, ham, hot dogs, sausages, salami, beef jerky, and canned meats.

The day after the World Health Organization came out with its report associating processed meats and red meat with colon cancer, the news coverage went wild. Media outlets didn't go wild encouraging everyone to quit eating red meat and processed meats. They went wild making light of the information.

First, let's look at how the World Health Organization developed its report. The research arm, the International Agency for Research on Cancer, consisted of twenty-two public health, cancer, and other experts from ten countries. Members reviewed eight hundred studies on cancer to arrive at their conclusions. This agency has been doing such reviews since 1971. As a surgeon who has operated on patients similar to the ones these experts utilized in arriving at their results, I take their findings very seriously.

For colon cancer, they reviewed studies that involved thousands of patients who had colon cancer to see if there was a correlation between what the patients ate and colon cancer. If a significant number of colon cancer patients ate a certain food, they placed that particular food into group 1. Group 1 was labeled definitely carcinogenic. The word *carcinogenic* means cancer causing. There was a definite connection between the food in group 1 and the development of colon cancer. Here is a summary of the five groups they used.

Group 1: definitely carcinogenic

Group 2: probably carcinogenic

Group 3: possibly carcinogenic

Group 4: not classifiable

Group 5: probably not carcinogenic

Members of the panel found "sufficient evidence" (their terminology) that processed meats such as hot dogs, sausage, and smoked ham cause cancer of the colon and placed them in group 1 (smoking and alcohol were also placed in group 1). They placed red meat in group 2, labeled probably carcinogenic.

Now that you know the medical side of the report, let's see how the general public was presented with the information. Then you can decide if you want to change your eating lifestyle to avoid these foods. Will you base your decision on the medical report or on how the media and general public responded?

The day the report came out, an article on the front page of *USA Today* quoted three individuals commenting on statements made by the medical organization. All three comments belittled the medical literature the World Health Organization had studied to arrive at its conclusions.

The first quote was from the president of the National Hot Dog and Sausage Council. She was quoted as saying, "Our reaction is that this is a huge and alarmist overreach to some weak data. We believe there is absolutely insufficient science to support this and that hot dogs continue to be a healthy part of a balanced diet."

The second quote came from a professor of nutrition who said, "The occasional frank is fine, [it is] a once-in-a-while food."

The third quote was from a professional baseball pitcher who stated that fans don't come to the park to watch what they eat. "That's why I love baseball and all sports—kind of a way to get away from reality and have fun. Terrible food's a part of it. It's not going to kill you."

Several questions come to mind. At the top of my list, Why would you put the World Health Organization and the

National Hot Dog and Sausage Council on the same playing field when you are weighing the health plan for your life? *USA Today* also ran an illustration that was labeled "How much is too much each day?" The drawing contained three items: one and one-fourth hot dogs, six thin slices of ham, and two and a half slices of bacon. It labeled them "approximate amounts of foods that will raise your health risks by 18 percent."

Raising your health risk by 18 percent should not be taken lightly. If I am operating on a patient and an artery starts bleeding, would I ask for a clamp that would secure the artery 82 percent of the time, causing an 18 percent risk? Or would I ask the nurse to quickly hand me a vascular clamp I know will work 100 percent of the time?

As a surgeon who has removed cancer from the colon, I see an 18 percent risk as a serious risk. The harmful correlation between certain foods and colon cancer tells me to change my eating habits. I hope it tells you to change yours also. Avoid the risk altogether by choosing the proper eating habits.

The more you learn about the impact various foods have on your body, the easier it becomes to make positive changes. Medical knowledge is a wonderful guide in helping you avoid the wrong lifestyles and adopt those that are healthy.

Think of the total cost of damaging your health versus the taste of what you want to put into your mouth.

▶ Action Steps

1. Avoid all processed meats for the next seven days.
2. If you are at your ideal weight, commit to limiting all snacks to either fruits or nuts.

PART 4

LIFESTYLE 3:

EXERCISE

10. The Importance of Exercise

Three Is Better than One

Exercise is the foundation of your new healthy life. Exercise reflects your commitment. It requires discipline. It reveals to your inner self how determined you are. Your exercise lifestyle is the lifestyle that reinforces the others. If you become disciplined when it comes to exercise, you will become disciplined in many areas of life. Don't deceive yourself concerning the importance of exercise.

Exercise is the most important of the three lifestyles because it ties everything together. If you exercise, you are much more likely to get to and maintain your ideal weight and also decide to eat healthy foods. The interrelationship of all three of the lifestyles is an important factor in your overall health.

Many medical articles provide statistics about people who exercise. They reveal powerful numbers showing the great benefits of exercise. But I read such reports between the lines because I know that people who commit to exercise are also the same people who commit to eating properly and maintaining their ideal weight. Exercise is the cornerstone holding up your other two lifestyles. If you exercise, you are telling yourself you are serious about your health. To commit to exercise is to commit to health.

As we have discussed, it is nearly impossible to lose weight and sustain the loss unless you eat right and exercise. The three lifestyles of weight control, food, and exercise are intertwined. They all work together. If you are doing one without the other two, the odds are against you that you will be successful. All three lifestyles work together to defeat the enemy that hinders your health the most: LDL cholesterol. None of the three lifestyles can stand alone. You can be an expert in one of them, but if you ignore the others, you will fail. Think of the three lifestyles as three ways you care for your car. What happens if you use the highest octane gasoline in your car's engine but never change the oil? You even buy additives to place into the gas tank to make the engine spark cleaner. You take care of the car's appearance and even buy special car wax to make the outside shine like new. But sooner or later, the engine quits because you never changed the oil. Everyone is going to say they can't imagine why your shiny car is not running anymore because you always took such good care of it. The car looks great, but the engine died because you left out one element that was essential to keep it running properly. You didn't change the oil.

Perhaps you have heard about a marathon runner who is at an ideal weight and is exercising to the max. However, at mile twenty, the runner grabs his chest, stumbles to the side of the road, and dies from a heart attack. The autopsy reveals blockage of the left anterior descending coronary artery (called the widowmaker artery). That artery had been in the process of becoming blocked for twenty years and finally closed off. The blood work shows markedly elevated LDL cholesterol. The runner had perfected two of the three lifestyles he could control. He exercised and was at his ideal weight, but his terrible eating habits caused his demise. Following two out of the three lifestyles won't give you the healthy body you desire.

The Facts

Do not fool yourself. Do not think you can take a pill, or an aspirin, or a supplement and reach the health goals you want to attain. The goal should be to get as young physiologically as possible and stay there. You want to develop the proper habits and keep them. Don't miss the one opportunity to live life to the fullest. The medical literature teaches what works and what doesn't. Magazine or newspaper articles that are slanted one way or the other will not give you the knowledge you need.

What the medical literature says about the importance of exercise is based on research and statistics. Individuals who exercise a certain amount are compared to those who don't exercise at all. Both groups are studied to see what happens. Does one group have more heart attacks than the other? Does one group lose more weight than the other? The groups may even be divided into smaller groups. For example, those who exercise strenuously and get their heart rates above 80 percent of their maximum for a thirty-minute period are compared to those who walk briskly for thirty minutes and get their rates to only 40 percent of their maximum. Such studies answer the question, Which is good, which is better, and which is best? The information in the following chapters will answer these questions. Then you get to choose which of the groups you want to be in.

Die Active

He looked to be in his sixties as he jogged down the beach on Grand Cayman Island. I had seen him many times before, but that day I decided to run along with him so I could ask about his exercise program. When I jogged up beside him, he stopped to talk. He was seventy-five and ran three miles down the beach Monday, Wednesday, Friday, and Saturday. "And then I have to run back," he pointed out. He rode a stationary bike for an hour and lifted weights the other days, "except Sunday. I don't exercise on Sundays."

He was Italian and had eaten a diet similar to the one recommended in this book all his life. He loved fish and ate a lot of vegetables and fruits as well as nuts. He liked pasta and ate cereal with lots of fruit almost every morning.

I congratulated him on his lifestyles and expressed admiration for his commitment. He just looked at me and said, "This is my life. This is how I live." But the best part of his story was when he told me someone had brought a complete health machine to the island several months before. "It cost me a few hundred dollars, but I took the test," he told me in his wonderful Italian accent. "I am seventy-five, but the machine said I am sixty-one. I am younger than I am." He flexed his arms and pulled his shoulders back as he made that last statement. "Most of my friends my age are old. They sit around and drink, play cards, and watch TV. Plus,

128

they're fat—most of them." Then he made the statement that caused me to admire him the most. He said, "I want to be active until I die."

He smiled and trotted off down the beach, waving with one hand without even glancing back. He may not know medically why he can say, "I am younger than I am," but he is doing what we all should be doing: exercising, eating properly, and sustaining an ideal weight.

The majority of people see exercise as a way of burning calories and losing weight. That is true, but the calorie count is much less significant than all the other benefits of exercising and, of equal significance, the dangers of not exercising. The chapters that follow explain both.

▶ Action Step

1. Decide on a specific activity you will commit to doing five or six days a week that will cause your heart rate to increase for a sustained period of thirty minutes. Options include brisk walking, jogging, biking, swimming, and racquetball. If you have a medical problem, check with your physician before you begin.

11. The Best Prescription You Can Fill

"Exercise Medicine"

If your doctor told you that you have high blood pressure and wrote you a prescription to get it down, would you take the medication? What if the doctor explained that high blood pressure is a common cause of stroke? Would you take the medicine to get your blood pressure down to normal? I don't know anyone who has been diagnosed with high blood pressure who has refused treatment. It scares them to death to realize that something is going on that could lead to a stroke.

Everyone I know opts to do something about their high blood pressure once it is diagnosed, but I know numerous people who do not exercise, who choose not to take their "exercise medicine" to protect their health. Being sedentary is as harmful to your health as having high blood pressure. Not taking your exercise medicine is as bad as refusing a prescription drug to improve your health.

I am hopeful that many people are sedentary or do very little physical activity because they just don't know the facts. They don't realize how dangerous it is to sit on the sofa and watch television rather than walk for thirty minutes after dinner or go to a gym after work. They don't know that doing anything active is better than just sitting.

I am equally hopeful that when such people read about the damage being done physically to their bodies and the ways they can avoid the dangers that come with not exercising, they will begin a new journey. They will commit to a specified time to take their exercise medicine five or six days a week. Exercise is good for cholesterol, good for blood pressure, good for the mind, and good for life.

If I could prescribe a pill to be taken five or six days a week that would extend someone's life expectancy approximately six years, I guarantee you I would run out of prescription pads from writing so many prescriptions. Exercise is that medication. And it's free. Start to think of your exercise program as taking your prescribed medicine five or six days a week.

Being Sedentary Can Be as Dangerous as Smoking

When researchers compare the life expectancy of someone who smokes to that of a sedentary individual, the results are similar. The problems associated with smoking and a sedentary life are also the same. The overall health of a sedentary person is no better than that of someone who smokes. Everyone knows the danger of smoking. However, people don't realize that many similar damaging processes result from being sedentary. The end is the same.

Yet individuals who don't exercise never compare their sedentary lifestyles to the lifestyle of someone who smokes. They may even pride themselves on the fact they don't smoke. Very few people think of not exercising as being harmful.

Heart Attacks and Strokes

Neither do most people correlate exercise with the prevention of heart attacks. They do not have symptoms of a heart attack, so they have no concern for prevention. But two-thirds of the time the *first* symptom of a blockage in an artery in your heart is a heart attack. Few people know this fact, nor do they ask themselves what could prevent this from happening.

The American College of Cardiology/American Heart Association Task Force of Practice Guidelines stated that after having a first heart attack at age forty or older, 23 percent of women and 18 percent of men die within one year. Those death rates jump up to 43 percent of women and 33 percent of men within five years of that initial heart attack.

So many people have had a heart attack, but it was just a "slight one," they say. "All the doctor had to do was place a stent." And they go on their way. They continue living the same lifestyles they always have. Most are at least a little overweight. Very few of them know which foods to avoid. And many are couch potatoes who watch television most of the evening and do not exercise.

There are other arteries in your body besides the heart that undergo the blockage process. The LDL cholesterol particles do not pick and choose which artery to get into. The brain has similar arteries to those of the heart. A stroke most commonly occurs when the blood supply to a particular part of the brain is suddenly halted. To me, a stroke is even worse than a heart attack. If you survive a heart attack, your mind is still clear and alert. If you survive a stroke, you are left with many possible problems.

Some of the worst patients I have seen are those who had a stroke and can't talk or walk or take care of their personal hygiene. If you survive a transient stroke attack (a light stroke that lasts only a few minutes before recovery), you have a five times greater chance of dying than someone who has not had a stroke. Five individuals who have had even a light stroke will die over the ensuing years, compared to one person dying who has never had a stroke. Plus, within the following five years, there is a 15 to 30 percent chance you will have some form of permanent disability due to a second stroke. Most strokes leave people with years of aftereffects. Six months after a stroke, 20 percent of survivors who are sixty-five or older have difficulty speaking, a third can't walk without assistance, and 25 percent end up in a nursing home.

If you look up the prevention plan developed by the American Stroke Association, you will see that it is similar to what we are discussing here: ideal weight and exercise.

Learn what you can do to help prevent either a heart attack or a stroke. Don't wait for "initial symptoms" to occur. As a matter of fact, don't wait for any symptoms. Most of the time you go to a physician because you are sick or have symptoms that need to be addressed. The doctor gives you medication or performs an operation to take care of your problem. The majority of Americans do not focus on prevention but wait until symptoms occur before taking action. Most do not know they can prevent the bulk of their symptoms by following three lifestyles, with exercise as a major player.

The Importance of Exercise and HDL Cholesterol

If you were to read only one sentence in this section on exercise, I would want it to be this one:

Exercise is one of two main factors in increasing your HDL cholesterol.

Take a minute to reflect on the role HDL cholesterol particles play in the health of your arteries. Even if your LDL particles are numerous and are getting into the walls of your arteries, the more HDL particles you have, the more police cars you have to haul off those LDL invaders. Your HDL level is profoundly related to preventing the blockage and inflammatory process in your arteries.

Exercise is significantly related to your HDL cholesterol. A review in the *Archives of Internal Medicine* showed that for every point you raise your HDL level, you decrease your chance of having coronary artery disease by 2 to 3 percent. Exercising thirty minutes a day for six days a week raises your HDL level approximately ten points. This is a linear, progressive process and begins within a two-month time period. The report concluded by stating that exercise is "highly significant" in increasing HDL cholesterol.

Studies in medical literature concerning exercise often compare people who are sedentary to people who perform different amounts and kinds of exercise. One such report caught my eye. It pointed out that if you can't walk a quarter of a mile in five minutes, your chance of dying within three years is 30 percent greater than that of someone who can make that timed walk.

A brisk daily walk for thirty minutes is a thousand times better than sitting on the couch. If you are sedentary, today is a great time to begin taking your exercise medicine.

▶ Action Steps

1. Set a specific time of day for the next five or six days that you will perform your exercise program. Put it on your calendar as an appointment with yourself for better health.

2. Remind yourself each time you exercise this week that you are taking your exercise medicine.

3. If you take a statin medication to *lower* your lethal LDL cholesterol, remind yourself each time you exercise that you are taking an exercise medicine that will *raise* your hero HDL cholesterol.

12. Building a Stronger Heart

There are two basic types of exercise. Aerobic exercise increases your heart rate and causes your heart to have to pump harder, resulting in strengthening of the heart muscle. Anaerobic exercise strengthens the basic muscles of your body. What weight lifting does to strengthen your biceps, aerobic exercise does for the muscle of your heart. Only exercise can strengthen your heart. And the more strenuous the exercise, the stronger your heart becomes.

If you are sedentary, even a brisk walk will increase your heart rate. As you continue to exercise, your heart muscle will become stronger, and you will need to walk faster to get the same increase in your heart rate. Before long, you will be trotting in order to get your heart rate up, and soon you will find yourself jogging or doing another type of more strenuous exercise.

If you don't have a regular exercise routine, the most important decision you can make in this moment is to set aside a specific time dedicated to exercising.

Finding Your Target Heart Rate

Studies have shown that a sustained increase in heart rate has the most positive effect on the cardiac muscle. They also show that you strengthen your heart the most efficiently by getting your heart rate to 80 percent of your maximum rate and keeping it there for a thirty-minute period six days a week. Begin measuring your heart rate as you exercise—either with a monitor or simply by taking your pulse as soon as you finish exercising. If you choose the latter, feel your pulse for a minute on the radial artery in your wrist or one of the large carotid arteries in your neck just beside your windpipe.

There is a simple formula for determining your maximum rate and 80 percent of that rate. To find your maximum heart rate, take the number 220 and subtract your age. To figure 80 percent, simply multiply the above result by .80. That is your target heart rate as you exercise.

The Benefits of a Strong Heart

As your heart muscle strength increases, your heart will pump more forcefully and will not have to beat as often to pump the same amount of blood. You can determine how strong your heart muscle is by finding out your resting heart rate, or how many times your heart beats in a minute while you are at rest. To find your resting heart rate, lie down and relax for about ten minutes. Then take your pulse. A normal resting rate is around seventy-two. If you plan your exercise properly, you will watch your rate decline into the sixties, then the fifties, and finally into the forties. The stronger your heart muscle, the lower your resting heart rate.

Remember when I told you about my visit to the Cooper

Clinic? They attached all kinds of devices to my chest and prepared me for a cardiac stress test. They had me lie down and then left the room. Ten minutes later, they came back in and said, "Are you alive?" I wasn't sure what they were getting at, but then they laughed and said, "Your resting pulse is thirty-eight." At the time, I wasn't aware of all the numbers concerning heart strength and resting heart rate, but I was happy when they explained it to me. "The stronger your muscle, the more efficient your pump is."

When you are sleeping and your strengthened heart is contracting forty times a minute versus the seventy-two times per minute of a heart that has not been flexed or toned, your heart has more rest time between beats. It has to work only a little over half as much as the weaker heart to pump the same amount of blood. Strong muscle fibers also do not need as much oxygen as weaker muscle fibers in order to contract. Therefore, less blood flow is needed to deliver the essential amount of oxygen to the muscle. This is similar to an automobile engine that gets thirty miles per gallon compared to a less efficient one that gets only twenty.

One more medical research point and we will move on. Researchers studied something called the index of oxygen demand. They took the top number in a person's blood pressure reading and multiplied that by their heart rate and came up with an indication of how much oxygen their heart muscle would use before it ran out of oxygen and quit working. They concluded that a heart with a strong muscle needs only about half the oxygen of a weaker, unexercised heart muscle.

I hope these benefits will help you see how important exercise is for your heart and will make it easier for you to get off the sofa and begin your journey.

The Key to Prevention

While exercise is most important to prevent a heart attack, it is important even after a heart attack. If you have had a stent placed in a heart artery or had a bypass operation, you need to know that exercise is significantly important following such events. The amount should be determined by your physician, but you need to get in a cardiac rehabilitation program that includes exercise.

The medical journal *Circulation* reported a study of almost five thousand patients who had a heart attack and found that when exercise was included in their rehab program, there was a 26 percent reduction in subsequent cardiac mortality. Even more significant was the finding that those who exercised reduced their risk of having another heart attack by 27 percent.

Yet the main objective is still prevention. Remember that 85 percent of Americans over the age of fifty have significant blockages in the arteries of their hearts without having any symptoms. There are things you should be doing right now to prevent an initial symptom from appearing. Exercise helps prevent heart attacks. Exercise motivates you to commit to eating properly to protect your arteries. And exercise helps you lose weight. Exercise is a key to prevention.

Find an Exercise That Works for You

If you were to ask me what exercise is best for your heart, I would tell you that anything that increases your heart rate works. That includes everything from a brisk walk to running three consecutive eight-minute miles. Swimming, cycling, racquetball—anything that elevates your heart rate and keeps it there for a thirty-minute period five or six days a week is good. If you were to ask me, a good elliptical machine or a treadmill or a membership to a nearby gym is the best Christmas present you could give yourself.

If you are completely sedentary, you may get your heart rate elevated to 80 percent of your maximum the first time you go on a brisk walk. The first step is to get your body moving, elevate your heart rate, and keep it there for a thirty-minute period. You will slowly progress and will need to work harder to elevate your heart rate.

If you are just starting to exercise, begin with a thirty-minute walk five or six days the first week. Then the second week try jogging (or slow trotting) for the first two minutes of your thirty-minute workout. You can gradually increase the amount of time you spend jogging—to four minutes, then six, and so forth—until you are jogging for the entire thirty minutes.

A study reported in the *Archives of Internal Medicine* involved twenty thousand men and women whose ages ranged from twenty to ninety-three. Two groups were involved. One group jogged and the other didn't.

The jogging group consisted of those who jogged between one and two and a half hours per week. Based on what we have been discussing, you can see this was not an extremely intense group of joggers. Instead of jogging thirty minutes a day six days a week, as encouraged above, these people jogged thirty minutes a day only two to five days a week. Nevertheless, they experienced some profound benefits.

1. They reduced their risk of premature death by 44 percent compared to those who didn't jog.
2. Jogging added 6.2 years to the life expectancy of the men and 5.6 years to the life expectancy of the women.

But other types of exercise can be just as effective. If you have joint problems, an elliptical trainer is a good choice. The machine is easy on your joints because the stride is smooth, with no pounding on your knees or hips. Also, your arms assist in the movement of the elliptical, so your legs don't have to do all the work. You may have to try several elliptical machines to find one that fits your body. Swimming is also a good choice for those with joint problems.

The bottom line is you can begin with any kind of aerobic exercise that is intense enough to elevate your heart rate. Just get started and expect your life expectancy to increase.

▶ Action Steps

1. Determine your maximum and your target heart rates.
2. Record your heart rate at the end of each thirty-minute exercise period for a week.
3. Record your resting heart rate weekly for the next three months.

Conclusion

I had an interesting discussion recently. I was on a scuba diving trip off the south coast of Cuba. Some of the most beautiful coral reefs you will ever see are located there. I was on a trip called a "live aboard," which means the divers live onboard a boat for a week. There were about a dozen divers, and of course we got to know each other very well.

Late one afternoon, we were sitting on the deck discussing the three dives we had taken that day. For some reason, one of the divers brought up the fact that he and his wife had a signed agreement covering when they would quit driving their cars when they got older. "We did it so our children won't have to make that decision for us. There will come a time when we are in a nursing home where we are taken care of, and we will prevent our children from having to make some hard decisions concerning us."

That sounded honorable—looking out for their children. But the conversation got worse. Two or three of the divers began talking about how bad it is going to be as they grow older. The conclusion was that health care is improving in the

United States and people are living longer. They were sure the last ten to fifteen years of their lives were going to be terrible. As the discussion continued, I couldn't help but think how true their conclusions were. I recalled hearing something on television: the most dreaded disease process we confront today is that of dementia. Parents, grandparents, and older friends are developing Alzheimer's disease. When I was young, it was called hardening of the arteries. There are two main types of dementia: Alzheimer's dementia and vascular dementia.

Vascular dementia is caused by a problem in the arterial system, the vascular system. The large arteries supplying the brain become partially blocked, resulting in less blood flow to the brain, or smaller arteries within the brain become inflamed or blocked.

With Alzheimer's dementia, plaque-like substances form in the brain tissue or tangles develop around the nerves. Medical literature reveals that there is a vascular component in a significant percentage of Alzheimer's cases.

Research on dementia as a whole has found that there is an arterial component to the majority of all the dementias. That is an exciting find because although there is no cure, there are definite steps we can take to help prevent the problem. The foods we eat are significant. Whether we exercise makes a difference. We should learn all the possible steps we can take to head off the most dreaded disease process we confront today in America.

My thoughts were interrupted as one diver's voice became louder and louder. I hadn't commented up to that point, but as I listened to what he had to say, I became more encouraged to do so. He said, "It has been shown that we are all going to live longer, and all the things we lived for are going to be for naught. We are going to end up being taken care of. The things we worked so hard to get are going to be taken away from us. We are going to live longer, but the extra years are going to be dreadful compared to how we are now living. We will end up living in an extended care facility and will have very little say concerning what we do. And one in nine of us will end up with significant dementia." He ended his lecture with something I couldn't let pass. He said, "And there will be absolutely nothing we can do about it."

I had to say something. "Let me tell you about an article in the *Journal of the American Medical Association.*" I had their attention. "Contrary to what most people realize, there are many things we can do to help prevent the scenario you are predicting." Everyone suddenly seemed very attentive.

"It is true that we are living longer. Modern medicine allows us to live longer than the generation before us. And many will end up exactly as you are predicting—inactive, unable to carry on and do the things they would like to do. As you say, one out of the nine sitting here will end up with dementia and will not be able to carry on a sensible conversation, unless . . . each of us begins doing something about it now. The one in nine prediction doesn't have to come true. To say there is absolutely nothing we can do about it is completely wrong." I then explained that the younger we get started with prevention, the better.

"After the age of fifty, you need to go by your physiological age rather than the number of years since you were born. You can turn your physiological age back seven to twelve years. It is not bad to live to be ninety if you can still get around like a seventy-eight-year-old." They remained attentive.

I went on to explain that it isn't the number of extra years we are going to live but the quality of those additional years that is so important. I gave them a few examples. One was of a man I know who is a well-known singer. I saw him not too long ago and told him I had always admired his singing, but the one thing I admired most about him was that he was caught speeding when he was ninety-four. (He blamed it on his wife. He told the officer she had been asking him a lot of questions.) My aunt Myrtle acted like a teenager well into her eighties. She would smile and tell me, "Why grow up if you don't have to?"

"It is not the number of years that is important but the quality of those years," I explained to them.

"What about the medical article you mentioned?" the diver who had said absolutely nothing could be done about dementia asked.

I began explaining the report. "It was a study of eighteen hundred individuals that covered a period of fourteen years. They were studied for Alzheimer's dementia. Here is what researchers found.

"What foods the people ate was the first topic. At one end of the scale were the people who ate the most meat and dairy. They were the ones who ate the most saturated fat. At the other end of the scale were the people who adhered to the fruits and vegetables and fish diet. Here is the conclusion: the ones who ate the healthy diet had a 40 percent less chance of developing Alzheimer's dementia."

I knew I had their attention because no one said a word. I continued.

"The second topic covered was exercise. At one end of the scale were the sedentary people, the couch potatoes. At the opposite end were the ones who exercised the most. Those who exercised the most had a 48 percent lower risk for Alzheimer's dementia." Still no comment from the previously talkative group.

"Lastly, they found a subgroup of people who did both—ate properly and exercised the most. People in this group were over 60 percent less likely to develop dementia."

When I finished my dissertation, I wasn't sure how this medical knowledge would sit with our group. The group was quiet, and we were called to dinner about ten minutes later. For dessert, we were served a chocolate pound cake with ice cream on top. I felt a little empowered when I noticed that three of the nine in our group passed up the dessert. I did have to wince a little when I saw the diver who said, "And there will be absolutely nothing we can do about it" take the dessert. I winced a little more when I saw he was the only one who scraped his spoon around the edge of his bowl to get the last drop of melted ice cream from the sides.

What Is Your Destination for the Rest of Your Life?

Fix this statement in your mind: the course you are on today determines your destination.

So many people think it is normal to add a couple of pounds a year. But you don't have to go up a waist size or a dress size each year.

Don't eat something just because it tastes good. Prove to yourself that you have the discipline to change your habits. Changing your habits changes your destiny. Eat well because you care about the rest of your life.

Don't be tricked into thinking you can eat anything you want in moderation and be healthy. That is what many say. Others say, "I'm just too tired to exercise." And so they retreat to the couch and watch television all evening and take pride in their occasional walk to the kitchen to find a snack. Is that what you really want?

The majority of people seldom reflect on their most prized possession—their health—until it is too late. They develop diabetes or high blood pressure or have a heart attack or a stroke. They do not realize they could have prevented such things. These people are living for the moment, not the lifetime.

At the same time, most people count on living longer. They have plans for the next cruise, the next golf game, the next grandbaby to welcome into the world, or the next wedding anniversary. All of us intend to live as long as we can. So why don't we live each day as though we want to live many more years in good health?

As we near the end of this book, think about this. You have two segments of life left to live: the present and the future. Look at them carefully and ponder what they actually mean.

The present. By developing proper lifestyles of getting to an ideal weight, eating the proper foods, and developing a personal exercise program, you can have a quality life in the present—today.

The future. This period is even more significant than the present. It involves the last ten or so years of your life. And you can actually look forward to those years with a sense of anticipation instead of dread. How? By changing course. If you are on the couch-potato course now, your destination will likely be dementia and dependency as you age. Is that what you want? I doubt it. Remember, dependency on others doesn't affect just you. It has a profound effect on your spouse, your children, your grandchildren. Future years are influenced by the choices you make today. They can be quality years or terrible years for you and everybody you know. What you do now in the present determines your destination in the future. It is your choice. By reading this book, you have learned how you can become younger physiologically than you are right now. If you change your lifestyles, you can be fifty physiologically when you are sixty-two chronologically. You can reset your physiological age by making life changes. Such changes will be worth far more than all the money you will ever have in your bank account. Switch courses now. Jump ship from average to exceptional and determine your destination by following the plan set forth in this book. Start today. Remember the formula: get to your ideal weight, avoid the bad foods and eat the good foods, and exercise. Don't let others tell you it is too hard. That is average thinking. Shoot for a better destiny. Your future depends on it.

Your future years are not set in stone. You are not destined to end life in poor health like so many others will. What we do begins with what we think. I like to rehearse a wonderful thought from the Book of Wisdom: "As [a man] thinketh in his heart, so is he" (Prov. 23:7 KJV). Let that be an encouragement to you as you begin thinking about the way you want to finish your journey. Dwell on it every day. Think about it at every meal. Before you know it, you will be living it in your heart, and it will empower your will. You can have vitality and remain active until the end. You don't have to just think about it; you can do it.

As you read the last pages of this book, I want to convince

you of this fact: you can add quality years to the rest of your life. My desire is that you will find something, large or small, that you can change for the better in the three lifestyles that are under your control.

Over the years, people have said to me, "My doctor has never discussed with me all the things you have shared in writing about my health." I would like to shed some light on why this is true. Physicians with long hours and busy practices cannot go into what has been covered in this book with every single patient. I have written this as though you are my patient and I am your doctor—a doctor who has taken time to review the medical literature for you and given details on how you can improve your health. I want you to understand the specifics and know how to apply them effectively so that you can remain as healthy as possible. I want you to be convinced that you can improve your health.

I encourage you to think about your personal health and most pressing concerns. Then reread the parts of this book that focus on what fits you personally. After your second or third read, I hope you will pass this book on to a friend and encourage them to adopt new lifestyles for better health. Think of giving this book to someone as giving a referral. I ask you to refer your "book doctor" to other "patients" I would otherwise not have the privilege of treating.

▶ Action Steps

1. Write the following stats on a sticky note and place it on your bathroom mirror:
   • 40 percent reduced their risk of dementia by eating properly

- 48 percent reduced their risk of dementia by exercising
- 60 percent reduced their risk of dementia by doing both

2. Eat fish for two meals this week.

3. Use olive oil.

4. Eat nuts for your snacks this week.

Epilogue

Let me tell you about a man who impacted my life in a significant way. I was on my first mission trip overseas. I had traveled to India to work in a mission hospital. I had requested from the president of a pacemaker company in America a donation of fifty pacemakers to take with me. I wanted to take them to a city that not only had no pacemakers but also had no surgeons who knew how to place them into a patient's heart. I planned to supply the pacemakers as well as teach the surgeons how to perform the operation.

I landed in New Delhi and quickly traveled to the mission hospital in an outlying city. As I walked the sidewalks of the town, I passed through massive crowds. The experience reminded me of trying to move through the mass of fans exiting a stadium just after the conclusion of a sports event in the States. But then my eyes drew me into the reality of life in India.

Along the edge of a sidewalk were small statues. Some looked like elephants; others had several eyes or multiple heads or ears. As I got closer, I noticed something odd. People had placed bits of food at the base of the figures. Then I understood that these were all different gods. I was astounded to think that people really worshiped gods made of stone. They had ears but couldn't hear, they had mouths but couldn't speak, they had eyes but couldn't see. Yet they were worshiped. In India, this is the people's way of life. People are born into such a culture and raised on the belief that worshiping such gods can alleviate their stress and bring them happiness.

The mission hospital had fifteen heart patients awaiting my arrival. Some had been admitted weeks or months before. What I hadn't planned on was that most of these patients were at death's door. Their heart condition was called heart block. Their hearts would beat only forty times a minute no matter how active they tried to become. The result was progressive heart failure. When someone is diagnosed with heart block in America, a pacemaker is immediately inserted, and the patient's problem is corrected. The patients awaiting me had had the problem for months, even years. Their hearts were in near complete failure.

The day I arrived I was informed that one patient had died earlier that morning. Another patient had experienced cardiac arrest several times before my arrival and arrested once more within the first hour after I got there. She immediately became my first case for surgery.

The two Indian surgeons of the hospital were appreciative, not only because I had brought the pacemakers but also because I was going to teach them to perform the procedure. But even more appreciative were the patients. They were the ones I received the greatest satisfaction from. These pacemakers were lifesaving devices for them. The gleam in their eyes and the smiles on their faces demonstrated their appreciation that they had been given another chance to live. I will never forget their expressions of gratitude.

One patient still stands out in my mind. During my medical career, I had never had a more appreciative patient than one elderly gentleman in his eighties. He knew he was at the end of his life if he didn't undergo a pacemaker operation. He thanked me daily. I will never forget him. He was always sitting propped up in his bed with extra pillows. Always smiling. Every time I entered his room he extended his hand and repeated the same words: "Thank you so much for saving my life."

The night before his discharge I went to see him. Once again he extended his hand and thanked me. I told him I knew he was being discharged the next day, and there was something I wanted to tell him before he left.

"You know how interested I am in your physical health." I took a seat on the small wooden chair by his bed. "I am also interested in your spiritual health."

"I want you to know I am a very spiritual man," he replied. "I know about Hinduism, Buddhism, Islam, and Christianity. I consider myself an expert on spiritual matters."

Without faltering, he spoke at least ten minutes about the religions of the world. I learned a great deal from him. As I listened intently, he pointed out that there is only one God and all religions simply worship the same God but in different ways. "You worship God in your way, and I worship God in my way," he said, "but all worship is ultimately to the same God." He was so authoritative.

"You know, doctor," he continued, "there is a wall completely surrounding this hospital." I nodded and wondered where he was going with this illustration. "There are three gates that allow entrance into the hospital for treatment.

There is the main gate out front but also two additional side gates." He swept his arm through the air, and I had the feeling he was talking to me as if he were giving instructions to one of his sons or grandsons.

"Now," he said, "most patients come through the main front gate. But if I had come in one of the side gates, you would have still put a pacemaker in me and saved my life. God and heaven are like that. There are many gates into heaven but only one God. You Christians say that the only gate into heaven is through the main front gate. But I am going to get there through one of the other gates."

He sounded so convincing, and I was unsure how to respond. I had discussed differences between Baptists and Methodists but never between different religions. I was stumped.

"What you are saying sounds right," I began, "but I don't believe it quite works that way." I looked directly into his face. "I will come back in the morning before you leave."

I couldn't wait to get to my room and get out my Bible and ask the Lord for wisdom on how to present this patient, this new friend, with the truth. If this were a medical problem, I could go to surgical textbooks or articles in the surgical literature and find the authority. This was a spiritual problem, and I knew where to go to find spiritual authority.

I recalled the words of Billy Graham that the best place to start reading the Bible is in the Gospel of John. I began with John 1:1 and read to John 3:16, which says, "For God so loved the world that he gave his one and only Son, that whoever believes in him shall not perish but have eternal life."

I knew what the verse was saying, but that was not the proper response to my new friend's outlook on God and heaven. I read further. After more reading, I got to a verse that jumped out at me. I knew that verse was the answer. I closed the Bible and went to bed.

The next morning I couldn't wait to get to the hospital to see my patient, who desperately needed the truth about the one true God. The old gentleman was propped up on pillows and waiting with the same smile and the same extended arm ready to shake my hand.

"Do you believe in Jesus?" I asked him.

"Oh yes," he said with delight. "Jesus was a great man. He was one of the greatest prophets who ever lived." He moved and placed his feet on the floor, taking a sitting position directly in front of me.

I pulled my chair a little closer and looked into his unshaven face and said, "Do you believe he was God's Son?"

He shot back his answer. "Yes, I believe he was God's son." I was stunned. But what followed made me realize he didn't really know who Jesus was. He continued. "I also believe I am God's son. I believe you are God's son."

Pressing the point, I responded, "Do you believe what Jesus said?"

"Yes, yes. Jesus spoke very profoundly many times."

Curiously, the old gentleman watched as I opened my Bible. I looked at him and said, "Let me tell you one statement Jesus made. It is from the book of John, the fourteenth chapter and the sixth verse. It begins with the words 'Jesus answered.'" I paused and looked up at him, explaining that what I was about to read to him was not something I came up with. It was not just an opinion of mine but something Jesus himself said. I continued with the verse. "'Jesus answered, "I am the way and the truth and the life. No one comes to the Father except through me."'" I closed my Bible and pointed to it.

"This is what the Bible records Jesus said about God in heaven. Jesus said he is the only way to God. Jesus said there is only one gate. Jesus is the door. Jesus is the way. This is what I believe. I do not know any individual I would put my faith in more than Jesus and what he said." I lifted my Bible where he could plainly see it and continued. "I also believe the Bible. There is no other religious book I trust concerning eternity more than the Bible. It is Jesus and the Bible. Whether you believe those two or you choose to believe something else."

He sat there in a moment of silence. I hoped he realized I was not trying to persuade him, that I was not preaching to him. I simply wanted to give him the facts out of the biblical literature and let him decide whether he accepted them or not. He finally spoke.

"I have never thought about religion like that before." His eyes wandered momentarily, and then he relaxed as he stood. He stretched out his arm as he had done so many times, and his face began to light up with his memorable smile.

"I will think about that." He paused. "I will think about that." His other arm went around my shoulder, and he pulled me close for a long hug as he whispered, "Thank you for saving my life."

From the time I walked out of his room, that gentleman's words have not left me. I prayed not only that he would leave the hospital with his heart beating effectively but also that he would find the assurance of heaven because he chose the right way.

I want the same for you. Medical literature, read and applied, can add quality time to your physical life. But the Bible is special literature that can change your spiritual life so you can spend eternity with the greatest of all physicians. This is my hope for you.

Medical References

Alzheimer Disease and Associated Disorders

"An Association with Great Implications: Vascular Pathology and Alzheimer Disease." 20, no. 1 (2006): 73–75.

Alzheimer's and Dementia

"Fourteen-Year Longitudinal Study of Vascular Risk Factors, APOE Genotype, and Cognition: The ARIC MRI Study." 5 (2009): 207–14.

American Heart Association

"Heart Disease and Stroke Statistics: 2004 Update."

American Heart Journal

"Does Exercise Reduce Mortality Rates in the Elderly?: Experience from the Framingham Heart Study." 128, no. 5 (1994): 965–72.

"Erectile Dysfunction: The Need to Be Evaluated, the Right to Be Treated." 150, no. 4 (2005): 620–26.

"Lifestyle Determinants of High-Density Lipoprotein Cholesterol: The National Heart, Lung, and Blood Institute Family Heart Study." 147, no. 3 (2004): 529–35.

American Journal of Cardiology

"Dietary Fiber, Lipids, and Atherosclerosis." 16 (1987): 17–22.

"Effect of Addition of Exercise to Therapeutic Lifestyle Changes Diet in Enabling Women and Men with Coronary Heart Disease to Reach

Adult Treatment Panel III Low-Density Lipoprotein Cholesterol Goal without Lowering High-Density Lipoprotein Cholesterol." 89 (2002): 1201–4.

"Effect of Alcohol Intake and Exercise on Plasma High-Density Lipoprotein Cholesterol Subfractions and Apolipoprotein A-1 in Women." 58 (1986): 148–51.

"Efficacy of High-Intensity Exercise Training on Left Ventricular Ejection Fraction in Men with Coronary Artery Disease (the Training Level Comparison Study)." 76 (1995): 643–47.

"Management of Sexual Dysfunction in Patients with Cardiovascular Disease: Recommendations of the Princeton Consensus Panel." 86 (2000): 175–81.

"Prevention and Management of Cardiovascular Disease and Erectile Dysfunction: Toward a Common Patient-Centered Care Model." 96, no. 128 (2005): 80–84.

"Usefulness of the Total Cholesterol to High-Density Lipoprotein Cholesterol Ratio in Predicting Angiographic Coronary Artery Disease in Women." 68 (1991): 1646–50.

American Journal of Clinical Nutrition

"Diet, Nutrition Intake, and Metabolism in Populations at High and Low Risk for Colon Cancer. Relationship of Diet to Serum Lipids." 40 (1984): 921–26.

"Dietary Cholesterol from Eggs Increases the Ratio of Total Cholesterol to High-Density Lipoprotein Cholesterol in Humans: A Meta-analysis." 73 (2001): 885–91.

"Effects of Dietary Cholesterol on Serum Cholesterol: A Meta-analysis and Review." 55 (1992): 1060–70.

"Effects of Two Low-Fat Stanol Ester-Containing Margarines on Serum Cholesterol Concentrations as Part of a Low-Fat Diet in Hypercholesterolemic Subjects." 69 (1999): 403–10.

"High-Monounsaturated-Fat Diets for Patients with Diabetes Mellitus." 67 (1998): 577–82.

"Hypocholesterolemic Effects of Oat-bran or Bean Intake for Hypercholesterolemic Men." 40 (1984): 1146–55.

"Individual Fatty Acid Effects on Plasma Lipids and Lipoproteins: Human Studies." 65 (1997): 1628–44.

"Mortality in Vegetarians and Nonvegetarians: Detailed Findings from a Collaborative Analysis of Five Prospective Studies." 70, no. 3 (1999): 5165–245.

"Plasma Lipoprotein Profile and Lipolytic Activities in Response to the Substitution of Lean White Fish for Other Animal Protein Sources in Premenopausal Women." 63, no. 3 (1996): 315–21.

"Plasma Lipoprotein Response to Substituting Fish for Red Meat in the Diet." 53, no. 5 (1991): 1171–76.

"Red Meat Consumption and Risk of Type 2 Diabetes: Three Cohorts of US Adults and an Updated Meta-analysis." 94, no. 4 (2011): 1088–96.

"Relation of Changes in Dietary Lipids and Weight, Trial Years 1–6, to Change in Blood Lipids in the Special Intervention and Usual Care Groups in the Multiple Risk Factor Intervention Trial." 65 (1997): 272–88.

American Journal of Epidemiology

"Physical Activity as an Index of Heart Attack Risk in College Alumni." 108 (1978): 161–75.

"Prospective Study of Alcohol Consumption Quantity and Frequency and Cancer-Specific Mortality in the US Population." 174 (2011): 1044–53.

"Total Cholesterol and High Density Lipoprotein Cholesterol as Important Predictors of Erectile Dysfunction." 140, no. 10 (1994): 930–37.

American Journal of Medicine

"Alcohol versus Exercise for Coronary Protection." 79 (1985): 231–40.

"Epidemiologic Aspects of Lipid Abnormalities." 105 (1998): 48–57.

American Journal of Surgery

"Surgery, Drugs, Lifestyle, and Hyperlipidemia." 169, no. 4 (1995): 374–78.

Annals of Epidemiology

"Lipids and Risk of Coronary Heart Disease: The Framingham Study." 2 (1992): 23–28.

Annals of Internal Medicine

"Sexual Function in Men Older than Fifty Years of Age: Results from the Health Professionals Follow-up Study." 139, no. 3 (2003): 161–68.

Annals of Neurology

"Dietary Fat Intake and Risk of Incident Dementia in the Rotterdam Study." 42, no. 5 (1997): 776–82.

"Dietary Fat Types and 4-Year Cognitive Change in Community-Dwelling Older Women." 72 (2012): 124-34.

Archives of Internal Medicine

"Effect of Aerobic Exercise Training on Serum Levels of High-Density Lipoprotein Cholesterol: A Meta-analysis." 167, no. 10 (2007): 999–1008.

"The Effect of Lifestyle Modification and Cardiovascular Risk Factor Reduction on Erectile Dysfunction: A Systematic Review and Meta-analysis." 171, no. 20 (2011): 1797–803.

"Effects of Low-Dose Niacin on High Density Lipoprotein Cholesterol and Total Cholesterol/High Density Lipoprotein Cholesterol Ratio." 148 (1988): 2493–95.

"Effects of the Amount of Exercise on Body Weight, Body Composition, and Measures of Central Obesity." 164 (2004): 31–39.

"Extended-Release Niacin vs. Gemfibrozil for the Treatment of Low Levels of High-Density Lipoprotein Cholesterol." 160 (2000): 1177–84.

"Lifestyle for Erectile Dysfunction: A Good Choice." 172, no. 3 (2012): 295–96.

"Prescribing Exercise at Varied Levels of Intensity and Frequency: A Randomized Trial." 165 (2005): 2362–69.

Archives of Neurology

"Use of Lipid-Lowering Agents, Indication Bias, and the Risk of Dementia in Community-Dwelling Elderly People." 59 (2002): 223–27.

Atherosclerosis

"Does Weight Loss Cause the Exercise-Induced Increase in Plasma High Density Lipoproteins?" 47 (1983): 173–85.

"Relationship between Physical Activity and HDL-Cholesterol in Healthy Older Men and Women: A Cross-sectional and Exercise Intervention Study." 127, no. 2 (1996): 177–83.

British Journal of Cancer

"Nutrition, Lifestyle, and Colorectal Cancer Incidence: A Prospective Investigation of 10998 Vegetarians and Non-vegetarians in the United Kingdom." 90, no. 1 (2004): 118–21.

British Medical Journal

"Alcohol and Cardiovascular Disease: The Status of the U Shaped Curve." 303 (1991): 565–68.

"Midlife Vascular Risk Factors and Alzheimer's Disease in Later Life: Longitudinal, Population-Based Study." 322 (2001): 1447–51.

"Risk of Death from Cancer and Ischemic Heart Disease in Meat and Non-meat Eaters." 308, no. 6945 (1994): 1667–70.

Canadian Journal of Cardiology

"Dietary Fiber, Complex Carbohydrate, and Coronary Artery Disease." 11 (1995): 55–62.

Chest Journal

"Effects of Exercise Training Amount and Intensity on Peak Oxygen Consumption in Middle-Age Men and Women at Risk for Cardiovascular Disease." 128 (2005): 2788–93.

Circulation

"Aerobic Capacity in Patients Entering Cardiac Rehabilitation." 113 (2006): 2706–12.

"Cardiovascular Implications of Erectile Dysfunction." 23, no. 21 (2011): 609–11.

"Clinical Cardiology: Physician Update: Erectile Dysfunction and Cardiovascular Disease." 123, no. 1 (2011): 98–101.

"Effect Size Estimates of Lifestyle and Dietary Changes on All-Cause Mortality in Coronary Artery Disease Patients: A Systematic Review." 112 (2005): 924–34.

"Exercise Prescription and Proscription for Patients with Coronary Artery Disease." 112, no. 15 (2005): 2354–63.

"Impact of Cardiac Rehabilitation on Mortality and Cardiovascular Events after Percutaneous Coronary Intervention in the Community." 123 (2011): 2344–52.

"An Overview of Randomized Trials of Rehabilitation with Exercise after Myocardial Infarction." 80 (1989): 234–44.

"Prevention of the Angiographic Progression of Coronary and Vein-Graft Atherosclerosis by Gemfibrozil after Coronary Bypass Surgery in Men with Low Levels of HDL Cholesterol." 96 (1997): 2137–43.

"Red and Processed Meat Consumption and Risk of Incident Coronary Heart Disease, Stroke, and Diabetes Mellitus: A Systematic Review and Meta-analysis." 121, no. 21 (2010): 2271–83.

"Reduction of Serum Cholesterol in Postmenopausal Women with Previous Myocardial Infarction and Cholesterol Malabsorption Induced by Dietary Sitostanol Ester Margarine: Women and Dietary Sitostanol." 96 (1997): 4226–31.

"Relationship between Erectile Dysfunction and Silent Myocardial Ischemia in Apparently Uncomplicated Type 2 Diabetic Patients." 110 (2004): 22–26.

"Relative Intensity of Physical Activity and Risk of Coronary Heart Disease." 107 (2003): 1110–16.

"Secondary Prevention by Raising HDL Cholesterol and Reducing Triglycerides in Patients with Coronary Artery Disease." 102 (2000): 21–27.

"Statement on Exercise: Benefits and Recommendations for Physical Activity Programs for All Americans: A Statement for Health Professionals by the Committee on Exercise and Cardiac Rehabilitation of the Council on Clinical Cardiology, American Heart Association." 94, no. 4 (1996).

"Third Report of the National Cholesterol Education Program: Expert Panel on Detection, Evaluation, and Treatment of High Blood Cholesterol in Adults (Adult Treatment Panel III) Final Report." 106 (2002): 3143.

Diabetes Care

"Can Adoption of Regular Exercise Later in Life Prevent Metabolic Risk for Cardiovascular Disease?" 28 (2005): 694–701.

European Urology

"Association between Smoking, Passive Smoking, and Erectile Dysfunction: Results from the Boston Area Community Health Survey." 52, no. 2 (2007): 416–22.

Federal Register

"U.S. Department of Health and Human Services Food and Drug Administration: Food Labeling; Health Claims: Soluble Fiber from Certain Foods and Coronary Heart Disease: Final Rule." 63 (1998): 8103–21.

Hypertension

"Benefit of Low-Fat over Low-Carbohydrate Diet on Endothelial Health in Obesity." 51 (2008): 376–82.

International Journal of Clinical Practice

"Endothelial Dysfunction Links Erectile Dysfunction to Heart Disease." 59, no. 2 (2005): 225–29.

"Erectile Dysfunction and Coronary Artery Disease Prediction: Evidence-Based Guidance and Consensus." 64, no. 7 (2010): 848–57.

"Past, Present, and Future: A Seven-Year Update of Sildenafil Citrate (Viagra)." 59, no. 6 (2005): 680–91.

"The Temporal Relationship between Erectile Dysfunction and Cardiovascular Disease." 61, no. 12 (2007): 2019–28.

International Journal of Impotence Research

"Dietary Factors in Erectile Dysfunction." 18, no. 4 (2006): 370–74.

"Erectile Dysfunction Association with Physical Activity Level and Physical Fitness in Men Aged 40–75 Years." 23, no. 3 (2011): 115–21.

"Erectile Dysfunction in Heart Disease Patients." 16, no. 2 (2004): 513–17.

"Mediterranean Diet Improves Erectile Function in Subjects with the Metabolic Syndrome." 18, no. 4 (2006): 405–10.

International Journal of Sports Medicine

"Comparison of Exercise and Normal Variability on HDL Cholesterol Concentrations and Lipolytic Activity." 17, no. 5 (1996): 332–37.

"Variability in the Response of HDL Cholesterol to Exercise Training in the Heritage Family Study." 23, no. 1 (2002): 1–9.

Journal of Alzheimer's Disease

"Vascular Risk Factors: Imaging and Neuropathologic Correlates." 20 (2010): 699–709.

Journal of Clinical Hypertension

"Therapeutic Effect of an Interval Exercise Training Program in the Management of Erectile Dysfunction in Hypertensive Patients." 11, no. 3 (2009): 125–29.

Journal of Investigative Medicine

"Cholesterol and Coronary Heart Disease: Predicting Risks in Men by Changes in Levels and Ratios." 43 (1995): 443–50.

Journal of Nutrition

"Impact of Non-digestible Carbohydrates on Serum Lipoproteins and Risk for Cardiovascular Disease." 129 (1999): 1457–66.

"Modulation of Inflammation and Cytokine Production by Dietary Fatty Acids." 126 (1996): 1515–33.

Journal of Nutrition, Health, and Aging

"Fatty Acid Intake and the Risk of Dementia and Cognitive Decline: A Review of Clinical and Epidemiological Studies." 4, no. 4 (2000): 202–7.

Journal of Sexual Medicine

"Adherence to Mediterranean Diet and Erectile Dysfunction in Men with Type 2 Diabetes." 7, no. 5 (2010): 1911–17.

"Dietary Factors, Mediterranean Diet, and Erectile Dysfunction." 7, no. 7 (2010): 2338–45.

"Is Obesity a Further Cardiovascular Risk Factor in Patients with Erectile Dysfunction?" 7, no. 7 (2010): 2538–46.

Journal of the American College of Cardiology

"Current Status of Cardiac Rehabilitation." 51 (2008): 1619–31.

Journal of the American Medical Association

"Alzheimer Disease." 287 (2002): 2335–38.

"Beneficial Effects of Combined Colestipol-Niacin Therapy on Coronary Atherosclerosis and Coronary Venous Bypass Grafts." 257 (1987): 3233–40.

"Cardiac Rehabilitation after Myocardial Infarction: Combined Experience of Randomized Clinical Trials." 260 (1988): 945–50.

"Effect of Lifestyle Changes on Erectile Dysfunction in Obese Men: A Randomized Controlled Trial." 291 (2004): 2978–84.

"The Effects of Running Mileage and Duration on Plasma Lipoprotein Levels." 247 (1982): 2674–79.

"Erectile Dysfunction in Obese Men." 29 (2004): 2467.

"High-Density Lipoprotein as a Therapeutic Target: A Systematic Review." 298 (2007): 786–98.

"The Lipid Research Clinics Coronary Primary Prevention Trial Results: Reduction in Incidence of Coronary Heart Disease." 251 (1984): 351–64.

"Meat Intake and Mortality: A Prospective Study of Over Half a Million People." 169 (2009): 562–71.

"Multiple Risk Factor Intervention Trial." 248 (1982): 1475–77.

"Physical Activity, Diet, and Risk of Alzheimer Disease." 302 (2009): 627–37.

"Physical Activity and Public Health: A Recommendation from the Centers for Disease Control and Prevention and the American College of Sports Medicine." 273 (1995): 402–7.

"Physical Activity and Risk of Stroke in Women." 31 (2000): 14–18.

"Women Walking for Health and Fitness: How Much Is Enough?" 266 (1991): 3295–99.

Journal of the National Cancer Institution

"Dietary Fat and Postmenopausal Invasive Breast Cancer in the National Institutes of Health–AARP Diet and Health Study Cohort." 99, no. 6 (2007): 451–62.

Journal of Urology

"Longitudinal Differences in Disease Specific Quality of Life in Men with Erectile Dysfunction: Results from the Exploratory Comprehensive Evaluation of Erectile Dysfunction Study." 169, no. 4 (2003): 1437–42.

Lancet

"Atherosclerosis Apo-Lipoprotein E and the Prevalence of Dementia and Alzheimer's Disease in the Rotterdam Study." 349 (1997): 151–54.

"Convergence of Atherosclerosis and Alzheimer's Disease: Inflammation, Cholesterol, and Misfolded Proteins." 263 (2004): 1139–46.

"Effect of Potentially Modifiable Risk Factors Associated with Myocardial Infarction in Fifty-Two Countries: Case-Control Study." 364 (2004): 937–52.

"Statins and the Risk of Dementia." 356 (2000): 1627–31.

Mayo Clinic Proceedings

"Erectile Dysfunction and Cardiovascular Disease: Efficacy and Safety of Phosphodiesterase Type 5 Inhibitors in Men with Both Conditions." 84, no. 2 (2009): 139–48.

"A Population-Based, Longitudinal Study of Erectile Dysfunction and Future Coronary Artery Disease." 84, no. 2 (2009): 108–13.

Metabolism

"Cholesterol Reduction by Different Plant Stanol Mixtures and with Variable Fat Intake." 48 (1999): 575–80.

"Effects of Low-Intensity Aerobic Training on the High-Density Lipoprotein Cholesterol Concentration in Healthy Elderly Subjects." 48 (1999): 984–88.

"Lipoprotein Subfractions of Runners and Sedentary Men." 35 (1986): 45–52.

"The Relationships of Vigorous Exercise, Alcohol, and Adiposity to Low- and High-Density Lipoprotein-Cholesterol Levels." 53 (2004): 700–709.

National Institutes of Health

"Clinical Guidelines on the Identification, Evaluation, and Treatment of Overweight and Obesity in Adults: The Evidence Report." (1998).

Neurobiology of Aging

"Vascular Risk Factors for Alzheimer's Disease: An Epidemiologic Perspective." 21 (2000): 153–60.

Neuroepidemiology

"Serum Total Cholesterol, Apolipoprotein E Epsilon 4 Allele, and Alzheimer's Disease." 17 (1998): 14–20.

Neurology

"Midlife Vascular Risk Factors and Late-Life Mild Cognitive Impairment: A Population-Based Study." 56, no. 12 (2001): 1683–89.

New England Journal of Medicine

"Effects of Exercise on Plasma Lipoproteins." 348 (2003): 1494–96.

"Effects of the Amount and Intensity of Exercise on Plasma Lipoproteins." 347 (2002): 1483–92.

"Exercise to Reduce Cardiovascular Risk: How Much Is Enough?" 347 (2002): 1522–24.

"Gemfibrozil for the Secondary Prevention of Coronary Heart Disease in Men with Low Levels of High-Density Lipoprotein Cholesterol." 341 (1999): 410–18.

"Light to Moderate Alcohol Consumption and the Risk of Stroke among U.S. Male Physicians." 341 (1999): 1557–64.

"Reduction of Serum Cholesterol with Sitostanol-Ester Margarine in a Mildly Hypercholesterolemic Population." 333 (1995): 1308–12.

"Regression of Coronary Artery Disease as a Result of Intensive Lipid-Lowering Therapy in Men with High Levels of Apolipoprotein B." 323 (1990): 1289–98.

"Steering Committee of the Physicians' Health Study Research Group: Final Report on the Aspirin Component of the Ongoing Physicians' Health Study." 321 (1989): 129–35.

"Trans Fatty Acids and Coronary Heart Disease." 340 (1999): 1994–98.

Preventive Medicine

"Erectile Dysfunction and Coronary Risk Factors: Prospective Results from the Massachusetts Male Aging Study." 30, no. 4 (2000): 328–38.

"The Multiple Risk Intervention Trial IV: Intervention of Blood Lipids." 10 (1981): 443–75.

Stroke: Journal of the American Heart Association

"Alzheimer Disease as a Vascular Disorder: Nosological Evidence." 33, no. 4 (2002): 1152–62.

"Atherosclerosis of Cerebral Arteries in Alzheimer Disease." 35, no. 11 (2004): 2623–27.

"Exercise and Risk of Stroke in Male Physicians." 30 (1999): 1–6.

"Leisure Time, Occupational, and Commuting Physical Activity and the Risk of Stroke." 36, no. 9 (2005): 1994–99.

"Physical Activity and Stroke Incidence: The Harvard Alumni Health Study." 29 (1998): 2049–54.

"Physical Activity and Stroke Mortality in Women: Ten-Year Follow-up of the Nord-Trondelag Health Survey." 31, no. 1 (2000): 4–12.

"Physical Activity and Stroke Risk: A Meta-analysis." 34 (2003): 2475–81.

"Reduction in Incident Stroke Risk with Vigorous Physical Activity: Evidence from 7.7-Year Follow-up of the National Runners' Health Study." 40 (2009): 1921–23.

Richard Furman, MD, FACS, spent over thirty years as a vascular surgeon. He is passionate about helping people prevent the problem that kills over half of all Americans. Furman is past president of the North Carolina Chapter of the American College of Surgeons, past president of the North Carolina Surgical Society, and a two-term governor of the American College of Surgeons. He is cofounder of World Medical Mission, the medical arm of Samaritan's Purse, and is a member of the board of Samaritan's Purse. He lives in North Carolina.